INTERNATIONAL PUBLIC HEALTH

Global Health

Series Editors: Nana K. Poku and Robert L. Ostergard, Jr.

The benefits of globalization are potentially enormous, as a result of the increased sharing of ideas, cultures, life-saving technologies and efficient production processes. Yet globalization is under trial, partly because these benefits are not yet reaching hundreds of millions of the world's poor and partly because globalization has introduced new kinds of international problems and conflicts. Turmoil in one part of the world now spreads rapidly to others, through terrorism, armed conflict, environmental degradation or disease.

This timely series provides a robust and multi-disciplinary assessment of the asymmetrical nature of globalization. Books in the series encompass a variety of areas, including global health and the politics of governance, poverty and insecurity, gender and health and the implications of global pandemics.

Also in the series

The Political Economy of AIDS in Africa
Edited by Nana K. Poku and Alan Whiteside
ISBN 0 7546 3897 9

Global Population Policy
Paige Whaley Eager
ISBN 0 7546 4162 7

International Public Health

Patients' Rights vs. the Protection of Patents

YVES BEIGBEDER
Webster University, Geneva, Switzerland

Routledge
Taylor & Francis Group

LONDON AND NEW YORK

First published 2004 by Ashgate Publishing

Reissued 2018 by Routledge
2 Park Square, Milton Park, Abingdon, Oxon OX14 4RN
605 Third Avenue, New York, NY 10017

First issued in paperback 2021

Routledge is an imprint of the Taylor & Francis Group, an informa business

A Library of Congress record exists under LC control number: 2003065710

Notice:
Product or corporate names may be trademarks or registered trademarks, and are used only for identification and explanation without intent to infringe.

Publisher's Note
The publisher has gone to great lengths to ensure the quality of this reprint but points out that some imperfections in the original copies may be apparent.

Disclaimer
The publisher has made every effort to trace copyright holders and welcomes correspondence from those they have been unable to contact.

ISBN 13: 978-0-815-38980-4 (hbk)
ISBN 13: 978-1-351-15544-1 (ebk)
ISBN 13: 978-1-138-35819-5 (pbk)

DOI: 10.4324/9781351155441

Contents

List of Presentations

Foreword

The central question in *International Public Health* is: how can we reconcile the organizing principles of the dynamic market economy – competition, private initiative and ownership – with meta-economic values and principles, with the search for the common good, with the respect for fundamental ethical and moral standards, and last but not least with solidarity with the weaker members of the community? The systematic and on the whole successful efforts undertaken to meet this challenge since the late 1940s have led to unprecedented freedom, economic prosperity and social promotion in the OECD countries. Today, in an increasingly open and interdependent world the challenge is to find the right balance not only at the national but also at the global level. As the history of the 20th century amply demonstrated, failure to meet this challenge (or even to recognize its importance) weakens social and political cohesion, and ultimately also undermines the market economy.

The last 50 years have witnessed an unprecedented progress of internationalization. The opening of borders, the freedom, the ease of movement of goods, services, ideas, technologies, and not least of people, have been a source and manifestation of the success of political communities. Closed societies, that have tried to isolate themselves from this general trend, were falling behind. International organizations, created at a time when the current degree of internationalization and worldwide cooperation were a distant goal in the future, have contributed to this development. In fact, it would be difficult to imagine today's globalized world without the work of international organizations.

One of the principal driving forces behind the worldwide trend of internationalization has been the systematic reduction of the role of governments in controlling cross-border relations. True internationalization implies the expansion of the relative weight of non-state, non-governmental cross-border relations in all areas. This does not eliminate the need for international organizations, but puts them in competition with other forms of interaction and cooperation, with the growing dynamics of direct relations among states without passing through universal or regional international organizations.

International Public Health is a careful and insightful analysis of the World Health Organization (WHO), one of the principal specialized agencies within the United Nations system with a clear non-political mandate, by one of the leading contemporary authors on international organizations. Yves Beigbeder, with a long list of distinguished publications in English and French in this field, brings to the analysis both the knowledge and experience of the former senior international civil servant that he used to be, and the objectivity and the sharp analytical tools of the scholar. This book, like his earlier writings on international organizations, is of interest for both the specialists and for the general reader. The clear exposition and the fluent style show a felicitous contrast with the heavy bureaucratic language of most publications by international organizations.

The study deals in an exemplary manner with three key interdependent issues that are likely to gain in importance in the years to come: *first*, the role and effectiveness of international organizations to improve people's lives; *second*, designing and implementing public health policies to fight major diseases; and *third*, the issue of cooperation or conflict between international organizations on the one hand, and large pharmaceutical companies, on the other hand, or in broader terms, the division of responsibilities between the public sector and business and the question who should bear the costs of international solidarity with the developing countries in the health area, the taxpayers or the shareholders. The book is highly topical at a time when the cost of medicine and in particular of the drugs to fight AIDS in the developing countries (an issue analyzed with great clarity and detail by the author) has become one of the most highly publicized controversies in the debate on globalization and has turned into one of the make-or-break issues in the World Trade Organization (WTO) Doha Development Round negotiations.

WHO, like the other major international organizations, has had its share of ups-and-downs in the perception by the public and of fluctuations in the consensus among the member countries on mandate, policies and resources. This study shows not only the complexities of the tasks and the need for support by the member countries but also the role of leadership and of the quality of management in the success or failure of international organizations to make a difference.

The massive expansion of the role of government, in both liberal and socialist societies, during the last hundred years was the result of both the growing complexity of the modern economy and society and of calls for a more active role of the government in securing the common good. However, the record has also shown, that attempts to entrust all power to the government were not only the hallmark of political and economic oppression, but also were a source of inefficiency and waste. This has been true also for the health sector.

The expectations towards international organizations as well as towards national administrations, have greatly expanded in recent years: the progress of internationalization has increased the need for efficient international organizations, yet globalization has also reduced the scope of the public sector and the resources of governments and their regulatory power in all areas. This has amplified the pressure to find innovative approaches to the issue of health combining the strengths of both government and of private initiative and private business.

Beigbeder shows the importance but also the limitations of the *Global Compact* between business and the United Nations, an initiative of UN Secretary General Kofi Annan. He welcomes the innovation and recognizes the need for a better understanding between the world organization and the private sector. For too long there has been a mutual misunderstanding and even hostility between the supporters of international organizations and the advocates of free markets and private enterprise. It is high time to break the vicious circle where those who are for closing the gap between the developed and developing countries are fundamentally suspicious of business and the market economy, and those who believe in economic freedom and private initiative see international organizations as another example of government interference.

Yet, there is and there has to be a distinction between the role of international organizations as the collective instrument of national governments, on the one hand, and private companies, on the other hand. The principal conclusion of the book is that whatever the current or future extent of the cooperation between WHO and business, this has not and is not likely to solve one of the principal problems of the developing countries in the public health area: i.e. the access of their population to affordable drugs. International organizations are a tool of intergovernmental cooperation. They are also a tool of solidarity and a tool for dealing with global problems. It is clear that there is a good case to be made that it is in the interests of the richer, developed countries to help the poorer, developing countries to improve public health. This is a political, economic and a humanitarian interest. The question is, whether the costs of this assistance should be carried by the pharmaceutical companies or by the taxpayers of the developed countries. While there is a need for a balanced approach – the record shows how difficult is it to find the equilibrium between the requirements of the public good and the growing pressures to reduce the resources available to carry out policies in the public interest.

Dr. Otto Hieronymi
Head, Program of International Relations and Migration and Refugee Studies,
Webster University, Geneva, Switzerland

List of Abbreviations

ACT UP	AIDS Coalition to Release Power
AIDS	Acquired immunodeficiency syndrome
APOC	African Programme for Onchocerciasis Control
ARV	Antiretroviral
ASH	Action on Smoking and Health
BAT	British American Tobacco
CVI	Children's Vaccine Initiative
CVP	Children's Vaccine Program
DAP	WHO Action Programme on Essential Drugs
DOTS	Directly observed treatment short-course
ECOSOC	Economic and Social Council
EPI	Expanded Programme on Immunization
EU	European Union
FAO	Food and Agriculture Organization of the United Nations
FCTC	Framework Convention on Tobacco Control
FDI	Foreign direct investment
GATT	General Agreement on Tariffs and Trade
GAVI	Global Alliance for Vaccines and Immunization
GIFA	Geneva Infant Feeding Association
GPPP	Global public-private partnership
GPV	Global Programme for Vaccines and Immunization
GRI	Global Reporting Initiative
GSK	GlaxoSmithKline
HAI	Health Action International
IARC	International Agency for Research on Cancer
IAVI	International AIDS Vaccine Initiative
IBFAN	International Baby Food Action Network
IBRD	International Bank for Reconstruction and Development
ICIFI	International Council of Infant Food Industries
IFPMA	International Federation of Pharmaceutical Manufacturers Associations
IGO	Intergovernmental organization
ILO	International Labour Organization
Infact	Infant Formula Action Coalition
IOCU	International Organization of Consumers' Unions
ISDB	International Society of Drug Bulletins
ISH	International Society of Hypertension
ITAC	International HIV Treatment Coalition
ITC	International Trade Center
JTI	Japan Tobacco International

MDR-TB	Multidrug-resistant TB
MMV	Medicines for Malaria Venture
MNS	Market News Service for Pharmaceutical Starting Material
MSF	Médecins sans frontières
MVI	Malaria Vaccine Initiative
NATT	Network for Accountability of the Tobacco Transnationals
NGDO	Non-governmental development organization
NGO	Non-governmental organization
NID	National Immunization Day
OCP	Onchocerciasis Control Programme
OECD	Organization for Economic Cooperation and Development
OEPA	Onchocerciasis Elimination Program in the Americas
PAG	Protein Advisory Group
PAHO	Pan American Health Organization
PATH	Program for Appropriate Technology in Health
RBM	Roll Back Malaria
R&D	Research and development
SKB	SmithKline Beecham Biologicals
STI	Sexually transmitted infection
TDR	UNDP/World Bank/WHO Special Programme for Training and Research in Tropical Diseases
TNC	Transnational corporation
TRIPS	Agreement on Trade-Related Aspects of Intellectual Property Rights
UK	United Kingdom
UN	United Nations
UNAIDS	Joint UN Programme on HIV/AIDS
UNCTAD	UN Conference on Trade and Development
UNCTC	UN Commission on Transnational Corporations
UNDCP	UN Drug Control Programme
UNDP	UN Development Programme
UNESCO	UN Education, Scientific and Cultural Organization
UNFPA	UN Fund for Population Activities
UNHCR	UN High Commissioner for Refugees
UNHCHR	UN High Commissioner for Human Rights
UNICEF	UN Children's Fund
USA	United States of America
WHO	World Health Organization
WTO	World Trade Organization
WWF	World Wide Fund for Nature

Introduction

The objective of international public health has been well defined in 1948 by the World Health Organization (WHO) as its own objective: 'The attainment by all peoples of the highest possible level of health'. Health has been defined, also by WHO, as 'a state of complete physical, mental and social well-being and not merely the absence of disease or infirmity'.[1] In 1977, the 30th World Health Assembly decided that the main social goal of governments and WHO should be the attainment by all the people of the world by the year 2000 of a level of health 'that would permit them to lead a socially and economically productive life'. This commitment was confirmed by the Alma Ata Declaration of 1978. In May 1998, the Assembly adopted a new global health policy 'Health for All in the 21st Century'.[2]

Public health is first a government's responsibility. Governments formulate and run their national health system, set up their public health infrastructure, manage state hospitals and dispensaries, adopt public health legislation, including intellectual property policy, decide on training requirements and ethical standards of medical and paramedical personnel, approve, register and control the use of medicines, set up national social security and other health insurance schemes. They authorize and control complementary private sector health institutions and insurance schemes. This responsibility, with variations between the respective domains of the public and private sectors, is that of all governments in all countries, rich and poor, industrialized, developing and least developed countries. A government's capacity to manage effectively and efficiently a national health system is of course dependent on the country's political, economic and social position, on its resources, on the political will of its leaders to assign resources to that often neglected sector of public programmes. The political and economic beliefs of the leaders, or their electoral platform, in a range between statist and liberal theories, affect decisions on the relative importance of the public and private sectors in the health domain. In democracies, governments cannot ignore public opinion and electoral concerns. They are also subject to pressures from national industrial and commercial groups, and from citizens' associations. Citizens of any country will turn on their political leaders to claim adequate health care.

However, health problems cannot be resolved and contained within national frontiers as the AIDS epidemic has shown: a need has emerged for common health policies, for joint efforts to prevent or fight epidemics, to set international standards with respect to biological and pharmaceutical products.

International cooperation in public health started in the second half of the 19th century, with the creation of international health institutions and a succession of international sanitary conferences. However, their main object was to protect 'civilized nations' from tropical diseases through a sanitary cordon. The activities of the World Health Organization, created in 1948 as a specialized United Nations agency, were to benefit all countries.

Built over the basic national structure of governments, the domain of international public health is currently shared among three constituencies, First the large group of intergovernmental organizations (IGOs), created and financed by governments, whose programmes are also decided upon and controlled by governments. The second group is that of for-profit transnational corporations (TNCs), whose visibility and influence has benefited from globalization. The third group is that of national and international non-governmental organizations (NGOs), a vocal and influential counter-power to governments, IGOs and TNCs.

The intergovernmental network

The network includes a number of UN institutions, the World Bank and the World Trade Organization at the global level, and a few transregional and regional organizations.

Global organizations

Within the 'UN family' of organizations, the World Health Organization should, in principle, have exclusive rights to be the leader in international public health for two reasons: first, its mandate is entirely within the domain of public health, while the programmes of other UN agencies or Funds are only related to health in part. Secondly, the Constitution of WHO assigns to the Organization the ambitious (and unrealistic) mandate 'to act as the directing and co-ordinating authority on international health work' (Art. 2 (a)). Was this part of an aborted attempt to create a world government with WHO as its Ministry of Health? Perhaps an internationalist blue-print, but world power realities have limited the political role of the UN, and specialized agencies have only remained as elements of wider networks in their respective fields.

WHO says that it has four strategic directions for its contribution to efforts to advance health at global and country level:

- reducing excess mortality, morbidity and disability, especially in poor and marginalized populations;
- promoting healthy lifestyles and reducing risk factors to human health that arise from environmental, economic, social and behavioural causes;
- developing health systems that equitably improve health outcomes, respond to people's legitimate demands, and are financially fair;
- framing an enabling policy and creating an institutional environment for the health sector and promoting an effective health dimension to social, economic, environmental and development policy.

In practice, WHO sets normative standards and provides technical advice and assistance on medical and other health-related matters. It has advocated a major change in health policy with the launch of Health for All in 1977. Following the successful eradication of smallpox, it is currently promoting the eradication of poliomyelitis, malaria and tuberculosis control and the fight against the HIV/AIDS epidemic. Negotiations for a framework convention on tobacco control are proceeding. It is also updating its model list for essential medicines. Several of its current programmes are carried out in partnership with other organizations with the involvement of civil society and the private sector.[3]

The UN Children's Fund (UNICEF) is both a partner and a rival of WHO. WHO initially opposed the creation of UNICEF and then tried to limit its activities by placing it within the UN secretariat under close supervision of the UN specialized agencies. When these attempts failed, WHO has accepted, at times reluctantly, the growing and more visible role of UNICEF in health programmes while insisting on WHO's leadership in public health policies. Children's health has become UNICEF's main programme. While WHO is concerned with the health of populations at all ages, UNICEF's mandate limits its role to the health of children, and by extension, the health of mothers. One of UNICEF's strengths is its high-profile and effective operational role at country level, filling a void left by WHO. WHO and UNICEF are currently partners in such joint programmes as the eradication of poliomyelitis, the Global Alliance for Vaccines and Immunization, the Joint UN Programme on HIV/AIDS (Beigbeder (2001)).[4]

The United Nations Population Fund (UNFPA) is not a rival to WHO. Its mandate complements that of WHO, and of UNICEF, in a politically sensitive field, that of family planning, a field in which both WHO and UNICEF have been reluctant to engage. UNFPA assists developing countries to improve access to and the quality of reproductive health care, particularly family planning, safe motherhood, and prevention of sexually transmitted infections (STIs) and of HIV/ AIDS. It provides access to high quality and affordable means of contraception and STI prevention, including condoms. Contrary to the charges propagated by US conservative groups, UNFPA does not provide support for abortion services.

The United Nations Development Programme (UNDP) helps countries in such broad areas as democratic governance, poverty reduction, crisis prevention and recovery, energy and environment, information and communications technology. UNDP is a partner in the Joint UN Programme on HIV/AIDS, a co-sponsor of the Onchocerciasis Control Programme and a member of the Roll Back Malaria Partnership (see Chapters 5, 6, 8). However, with decreasing resources, it is a small actor in the health sector.[5] Its main potential influence in the health field has been applied at country level through the resident coordinator system. The Resident Coordinator, formerly a UNDP staff member, now serves as the designated representative of the UN Secretary General for development operations in the field, as well as being the designated leader of the UN country team in non-conflict areas. Through his/her direct access to the country's government head, and his/her coordination functions with all the UN agencies, funds and other bodies working at the country level, UNDP may have a direct impact on a country's health programme.

The creation of the Joint United Nations Programme on HIV/AIDS (UNAIDS) in January 1996, brought evidence of the lack of confidence in WHO's abilities to tackle the main health, social and economic issues of the AIDS epidemic on the part of the other UN organizations and the main donors. UNAIDS is a small umbrella organization drawing together UNICEF, UNDCP, UNDP, UNFPA, UNESCO, WHO, the World Bank[6] (see Chapter 5).

The involvement of the International Bank for Reconstruction and Development (IBRD, or World Bank) in health was not obvious. Its formal mandate is to provide financial capital to assist in the reconstruction and development of member states. Its current aim is to reduce poverty in middle-income and creditworthy poorer countries by promoting sustainable development through loans, guarantees, and non-lending – including analytical and advisory – services. The World Bank started giving assistance in the health sector in the 1980s, emphasizing the role of health programmes in poverty alleviation. International development goals now include reducing infant, child and maternal mortality rates, providing access to reproductive health care to all who require it. Cumulative lending by the World Bank to health (population, health, nutrition) projects have risen since the mid-1980s to about $11 billion over a 15-year period. New lending by the Bank in 2002 was at the level of $11.5 billion, of which $1.38 billion went to health projects, including over $300 million for support to HIV/AIDS projects.[7]

In financial terms, the Bank's assistance in public health exceeds WHO's total resources, which makes the Bank the largest single source of international financing for health. More importantly, while the Financial Institutions, the World Bank and the International Monetary Fund are specialized agencies of the United Nations, their nature is different. They cooperate with the UN and UN organizations but do not accept UN coordination or leadership. While the governance of UN organizations is based on the one country/one vote system, the Bank links voting power to members' capital subscriptions, in turn based on relative economic strength. As a consequence, rich countries under US leadership determine the Bank's policies, while UN organizations give more weight to the concerns of developing countries, the majority of their member states. The Bank's critics point to the Bank's history of secrecy, emphasis on free-market strategies, its ideology of decreasing the role of government in public health interventions and health care delivery. For these critics, the Bank places most responsibility for health on individuals, minimizes corporate responsibilities and health risks caused by industries, contributing indirectly to the unleashing of market forces in order to maximize profits for Western transnational corporations such as pharmaceutical companies and agrobusinesses. Through WHO's cooperation with the Bank – WHO providing technical expertise and the Bank, financial resources – WHO risks being associated with the Bank's ideology, privileging the role of the market in the provision of health and pensions, to the benefit of transnational corporations (Armada et al. (2001)). It also raises the issue as to whether the Bank intends to replace WHO as the leader in the field of international health. The Bank has already claimed to have sharper expertise in health economics and health sector reform than WHO (WHO (1996)).

In 2001, WHO was granted observer status on the World Trade Organization's (WTO's) Council for Trade-Related Aspects of Intellectual Property Rights, enabling WHO to monitor discussions on access to patented drugs. It also has observer status on the WTO Committee on Sanitary and Phytosanitary Measures and the Committee on Technical Barriers to Trade. More open trade and more accessible markets, WTO's main objective, have a direct effect on health and have rarely benefited the populations of poor countries. At the Doha Conference of the WTO held in November 2001 and later (see Chapter 4), the conflict between, on the one hand, international trade agreements, the protection of patents, and, on the other hand, the protection of public health and the access to low-cost, safe and effective essential medicines became public and made WHO's intervention necessary. WTO agreements also shape national policies and regulations on food safety, trade on tobacco products. Negotiations launched in 2000 to further liberalize trade in services will open health services markets to foreign competition, which may, in turn, worsen equity in financing and reduce access to care for the poor. In its relations with WTO, WHO finds itself in the difficult position of trying to plead for the interests of developing countries, while WTO, and similarly the World Bank, tend to place economic liberalization above health concerns for poor countries.

Transnational and regional organizations

As these organizations are not included in depth in the present study, only brief comments are given hereunder on a few selected organizations.

The Organization for Economic Cooperation and Development (OECD) groups 30 member countries from North and Central America, Europe and the Asia-Pacific area, countries sharing a commitment to democratic government and the market economy. It has active relationships with some 70 other countries, NGOs and civil society. It is best known for its publications and statistics, its main work focusing on its member countries. Through its Development Assistance Committee, it evaluates its members' development policies. In the development of health policies, the OECD has been described as a facilitator, whose influence comes from the value of its analyses and the influence of its networks. In an OECD Conference on Biotechnology for Infectious Diseases held in October 2002, participants agreed that, as OECD countries lead the research, development and production of new vaccines, they have a responsibility to build public/private partnerships between governments, charitable foundations and bio/pharmaceutical industries in developed and developing countries. These partnerships should allow researchers to find cures, pharmaceutical companies to make the profits their shareholders demand and help developing countries build the capacity and infrastructure to provide their citizens with the medications they need.

The European Union (EU), currently with its 15 member states, is involved in health policies through research funding, support and collaboration in the development of health systems and public health policies, and emergency assistance. With the 1991 Maastricht Treaty on European Union, it has acquired a new competence in public health in three areas: disease prevention and research, health information and education and the incorporation of health protection requirements in the EU's other policies. The Maastricht Treaty requires that EU policies towards developing countries should take into account development cooperation objectives.

As for the OECD, the 'Club of rich countries', EU members' economic interests tend to prevail over equitable health policies for developing countries in such areas as pharmaceutical, tobacco and agricultural trade policies.

For the record, the Pan American Health Organization serves as the WHO Regional Office for the Americas, covering 35 member states in North, Central and

South America. Its policies follow those of the WHO, as adopted by the World Health Assembly.

Transnational corporations (TNCs) and foundations

Public health is dependent not only on legislation, public institutions and state resources, but also on the private sector. There are state hospitals and dispensaries, but also private clinics. Fighting malaria, tuberculosis, AIDS requires effective medicines produced by private laboratories, which also carry out research and development of new drugs. Effective vaccines are the essential tool for the prevention of illnesses, such as flu or poliomyelitis. Pharmaceuticals account for 25 to 40 percent of a developing country's health expenditure. The pharmaceutical industry is therefore a powerful and indispensable actor in national and international public health.

Most large pharmaceutical companies are located in industrialized countries and sell their products internationally. The companies enjoy support from their own government as a profitable element of national economy, with a supportive network of doctors and pharmacists. They lobby effectively governments in order to influence national legislation, and, at the international level, to support, change or prevent decisions or recommendations of the World Bank, WTO, OECD, WHO and other IGOs.

The International Federation of Pharmaceutical Manufacturers Associations (IFPMA) has been admitted into official relations with WHO since 1971. Its membership of 57 manufacturers associations include virtually the totality of international research-based pharmaceutical companies producing the main brand-name drugs. It collaborates with WHO in drug quality consultations, influenza vaccine formulas, polio, the Children's Vaccine Initiative, family and reproductive health, substance abuse. Some of IFPMA's members have opposed the formulation of national drug policies in developing countries and the promotion of generic drugs, showing a basic contradiction between the aims of profit-making firms and those of WHO in its essential drugs policy. A few manufacturers have reduced prices of AIDS drugs in several developing countries under public pressure from NGOs (see Chapters 4 and 5).

The pharmaceutical firms SmithKline Beecham and Merck & Co. have joined governments, WHO, UNICEF, the World Bank and other partners to eliminate lymphatic filiarisis. Merck & Co. has donated ivermectin for large-scale treatment of onchocerciasis (river blindness) in a large programme coordinated by WHO, with FAO, UNDP, the World Bank and numerous NGOs (see Chapter 6). Aventis Pasteur and De Beers are partners with governments, WHO, UNICEF and others in the international coalition set up to eradicate poliomyelitis (see Chapter 7).

Transnational baby food companies have fought against the adoption, under WHO and UNICEF auspices, of the International Code of Marketing of Breast-Milk Substitutes in 1981. NGOs have documented and publicized violations of the Code by companies since then (see Chapter 3).

WHO and other UN organizations (as well as governments) increasingly enter into public/private partnerships in public health (see Part III). This raises the issue of the compatibility of private (profit-making) and public (general interest and health of the population) values and interests between the strong TNCs and the weak UN agencies. May guarantees be obtained that such ventures will not end in a domination of the former over the latter?

Another recent phenomenon is the granting of donations for health programmes by philanthropic US-based, business-related foundations. For instance, the William H. Gates Foundation, co-founded by Bill Gates and his wife Melinda Gates, focuses on child and maternal health in developing countries. In 1998 the Foundation gave more than $200 million to health-related causes, including $100 million towards children's vaccines, $50 million to prevent maternal and child mortality and $25 million to develop an AIDS vaccine. It awarded in 1999 $10 million to the UNDP/ UNFPA/WHO/World Bank Special Programme of Research Development and Research Training in Human Reproduction. The United Nations Foundation, created by Ted Turner, has given or pledged nearly $50 million to WHO programmes, also in 1999. Rotary International is an active partner in the global initiative to eradicate poliomyelitis, together with the UN Foundation and the Gates Foundation (see Chapter 7). Philanthropy is well-entrenched in US culture. While these donations have an obvious aspect of public relations, unattached, unconditional funds are always welcome to individuals and organizations who carry out the work.[8]

The counter-power of non-governmental organizations (NGOs)

Leaving aside business-related, profit-making organizations, NGOs, as voluntary non-profit organizations, make a substantial contribution to national and international public health. The retrenching of state and public responsibility in this area, consonant with economic liberalism theories, have increased their role, as cheaper and, hopefully, more efficient alternatives to governmental delivery systems. Their role may be generalized as three overlapping spheres (Koivusalo and Ollila, 1997:98):

- advocacy, lobbying and vigilance (policy and rights);
- provision of services on specific areas of research, counselling and technical support (knowledge and resources);
- providing global 'poverty' services in terms of relief, welfare and service provision in health care and population policies (services and charity).

At the community, local and national levels, NGOs support or prod their government into action, and/or provide services adding to or replacing state services. At the international level, NGOs lobby and challenge governments, IGOs, TNCs. They advocate better policies, launch campaigns, form coalitions, carry out research, provide services either directly or through local NGOs. They mobilize public opinion both internally and across state boundaries, they collect funds. Independent researchers, lawyers and scholars contribute theoretical arguments, scientific or empirical evidence to buttress NGOs campaigns (Weiss & Gordenker (1996). Among the main activist NGOs in the health field, The International Baby Food Action Network (IBFAN) consists of public interest groups working to reduce infant and young child morbidity and mortality. The Network vigorously supported the adoption of the International Code of Marketing of Breast-Milk Substitutes. It now monitors and publicizes the compliance (or non-compliance) of infant food producers with the Code. Infact, a national grassroots corporate watchdog organization, is best known for its successful Nestlé Boycott Campaign, also linked with the negotiation and implementation of the Code. Infact and Corporate Europe Observatory are members of the Network for Accountability of Tobacco Transnationals (NATT), which includes 76 NGOs from 51 countries working for a strong, enforceable Framework Convention on Tobacco Control (see Chapters 3 and 10).

A few NGOs, better known for their operational assistance work, have turned, in part, to advocacy on health issues. Médecins Sans Frontières (MSF) has launched in 1999 its Access to Essential Medicines Campaign. MSF is coordinating a strategy to implement the WTO Doha Declaration. In February 2001, Oxfam launched its *Cut the Cost* campaign aiming at reducing the price of vital medicines and allowing poor countries to bargain for lower prices with the pharmaceutical companies in order to have access to cheaper generic drugs. Save the Children has participated in the WHO-NGO Roundtable on Pharmaceuticals held in 1991. It holds strong views on the need for safeguards of WHO independence in its interaction with commercial enterprises. Health Action International (HAI), a global network of health, development, consumer and other public interest groups in more than 70 countries works for a more rational use of medicinal drugs. HAI represents the interests of consumers in drug policy. It campaigns for better control on drug promotion and the provision of balanced, independent information for prescribers and consumers.

Human Rights NGOs also deal with public health issues. Human Rights Watch supports the right of WTO member states to promote universal access to essential medicines, and the flexibility afforded to states by the Doha Declaration to relax patent protection, and thus lower drug prices, in times of public health emergency (see Chapter 4).

In early 2003, there were 189 international NGOs in official relations with WHO. Only a few of those could be described as 'activists'. Most of them, such as health-related associations, medical, biologist, dental, nursing and midwives associations, sanitary and environmental groups, and those concerned with a specific illness (cancer, diabetes, leprosy, trachoma) provide expertise, research capacity, financial resources without need for advocacy and confrontation.

Conclusion

There is no 'one voice' in international public health, which raises problems of legitimacy, coordination and effectiveness. At the national level, each country is sovereign in its decisions on health policy, trade, patents through its legislation and practice. However, many developing countries have weak institutions and are more exposed to external political and trade pressures than rich countries. Among the latter, the USA, the political, military and economic super-power is, currently, the uncontested leader in promoting open trade, the law of the market, the right of private enterprises to sell freely in foreign countries, the opposition to binding international regulation, the determination to ensure the strict protection of patents.

Other rich countries generally follow US lead in order to protect their own pharmaceutical industry, although not necessarily its insistence on the free trade dogma. Scandinavian countries retain a principled position as genuine advocates of the rights of developing countries' populations.

In the UN organizations, with the one-country/one vote system, developing countries have a chance to voice their problems and oppose measures not conducive to their population's health. However, decisions taken by the governing bodies of these organizations are influenced by the power of the rich countries, themselves subject to the effective lobbying of TNCs with their strong industrial and commercial weight. While the UN organizations cannot renege on their global obligations to serve all countries and their peoples, they are often placed in the ambiguous position of a powerless referee between pressures from consumers and other NGOs on the one hand, and rich countries and TNCs on the other.

The position in the World Bank, WTO and OECD is clearer: rich countries have a majority in these pro-free trade organizations. TNCs exert a strong influence within their international secretariats and in negotiations with governments, without the internal counter-weight of NGOs.

Although WHO was created as the directing and coordinating authority on international health work, it is now rivaled in this area by the World Bank with its larger funding, UNICEF with its higher visibility, and in specialized domains, UNFPA and UNAIDS. Even the UN, not WHO, and the G8 have recently launched the Global Fund to fight AIDS, Tuberculosis and Malaria. WTO's role in negotiating global trade rules has a direct impact on such issues as the access and affordability of essential drugs, food safety, the tobacco trade etc.

Still, WHO is the organization best-placed to collect the expert opinions and advice of high-level, independent international experts on public health and medical questions and to adopt policies reflecting a balanced international position. WHO should retain its status as the international authority on public health policy.

The legitimacy of TNCs is based on their business achievements and the satisfaction of their shareholders.

The legitimacy of NGOs has been questioned. Unlike political leaders in democratic countries, NGOs and their leaders are not elected by the people, they are self-created and self-appointed. Secondly, most of the major NGOs are based in North America and Western Europe and therefore do not abide by the 'equitable geographical distribution' factor prevalent in UN organizations. Their legitimacy relies on their values, themselves based on international conventions and treaties, including human rights instruments, the Geneva Conventions, the ILO Conventions, WHO policies and other international standards which have a quasi-universal recognition.

Coordination mechanisms within the UN system are still a 'work-in-progress' with considerable obstacles created by individual organizations and funds. Competition of organizations over visibility and funding often prevails over coordination and effectiveness. The financial organizations agree to cooperate with UN agencies, but do not accept their leadership nor coordination.

Can WHO coordinate public health programmes? WHO has no such formal or practical authority. At the international level, WHO has to prove its technical competence and capacity in order to convince its partners, case by case, that it is in the best position to assume such a role.

At the national level, only governments can coordinate international assistance. They have the difficult task of deciding which health programmes will have priority and which national and international organizations will give assistance or carry them out.

Large international NGOs are fiercely independent: they recognize no leader among them, nor would they agree to be coordinated by a UN agency.

Coordination in the public health field, as in most other international programmes, remains a voluntary effort, thus limiting the effectiveness of international health work.

Scope of the book

Both the United Nations and WHO have recently admitted the private sector as a new partner, besides their rulers, the governments, and their long-standing associates, the NGOs. In the domain of international public health, the formal recognition of for-profit organizations as legitimate actors raises the question of the extent and limits of the permissible interaction of WHO with these organizations in formulating recommendations and making decisions. Most governments have defined the role of the private sector in national public health in their own countries through legislation and regulation. In the wider and less structured world of international public health, rules and practices to be applied to the interaction between IGOs such as WHO and UNICEF, on the one hand, and industrial and commercial enterprises on the other, are still in the making. The main object of this book is to weigh the costs and benefits of this 'new partnership' or alliance, to assess the compatibility of the global mandate of the UN organizations concerned with public health with the profit objectives of business firms, to set possible limits to their interaction.

The book reviews specific international public health issues and programmes from the vantage viewpoint of WHO, which, in spite of its weaknesses, remains the key global actor in this domain. The interaction of WHO and other IGOs with profit-making enterprises, business-issued foundations and international NGOs as monitors, critics and advocates, will be reviewed.

Part I of this book sets the scene: the launching of the Global Compact by Kofi Annan, the UN Secretary-General, has opened the UN to business, as a key element of civil society, to the consternation of many NGOs (Chapter 1). Has the UN gone overboard in opening its doors to 'big business' without adequate precautions? Can the organization's programmes benefit from this association, without the UN losing its soul? Should the concept and functioning of the Global Compact be re-considered?

Similar hopes and concerns have been voiced when Dr Brundtland, the former WHO Director-General, opened her organization to the private sector more broadly and openly than before (Chapter 2). Effective medicines, vaccines and medical technology and materials are essential to public health: WHO needs to cooperate with the pharmaceutical industry, its researchers and producers. However, the industry has not extended its research on illnesses prevalent in developing countries, while WHO's programmes give priority to these countries. Has WHO clearly defined the boundaries of its relationships with the politically and economically powerful 'big pharma' and other for-profit firms, in order to protect its own identity and integrity?

The following Chapters give examples of WHO's consultation and cooperation with 'for-profit organizations' in specific areas and assess their results.

The first category (Part II) involves the setting of policies by WHO, generally with the support of NGOs, which have been opposed by private sector firms or industries. This has placed WHO in the uncomfortable position of being the target of NGOs for not being forceful enough, and the target of TNCs for threatening their interests. Chapter 3 deals with the promotion of breast-feeding, Chapter 4 with essential drugs and the pharmaceutical industry, Chapter 5 with the global HIV/ AIDS epidemic.

The second category includes Public-Private Partnerships for Health, which have flourished especially during Dr Brundtland's mandate (Part III). Questions raised: why these partnerships? Is international public health a beneficiary or a loser in these alliances? Chapter 6 reviews the first business partnership, the onchocerciasis control programme, Chapter 7, the eradication of poliomyelitis, Chapter 8, malaria and tuberculosis control programmes, and Chapter 9, the Global Alliance for Vaccines and Immunization.

The third category (Part IV) refers to WHO's rejection of cooperation with an industry, the tobacco industry, whose product is known to cause illness and death. In this case, WHO's policy is generally agreed by most Member States and strongly supported by NGOs. The public health enemy is named and the policy is not only non-cooperation, but a public fight against the industry (Chapter 10).

A Conclusion will try to strike a balance between the exigencies of international public health, the mandate of WHO and the need to maintain productive relationships with the health-related industry and business firms.

Should WHO be more selective in associating itself with business firms? Should it ensure that these firms give allegiance to WHO's objectives and policies, accept its role 'as directing and coordinating authority' in international public health work, follow its technical guidance and accept its evaluations?

Should WHO adopt an advocacy position in debates on intellectual property rights and access to essential medicines, or stand above the disputants as an arbiter? Should WHO press governments and WTO for a 'health exception' in trade negotiations and agreements?

Research for this book is based on relevant literature, books, articles, official documentation and press releases of IGOs, electronic searches of NGOs sites, industry sites, interviews with UN and WHO officials or retired officials. The texts of a few Chapters have been reviewed by WHO, UNICEF or foundations' officials, who are herewith thanked for their willing assistance. The editing skills of Mandy Eggleston are gratefully acknowledged.

Finally, the author has written this book in a personal capacity and assessments are his own responsibility – they do not necessarily reflect the views of, nor commit in any way, WHO and the other organizations referred to in the following Chapters.

Notes

1   WHO Constitution, Preamble and Art. 1.
2   The Declaration of Alma-Ata is in WHO *Health for All Series*, No. 1.
3   WHO's budget for 2000–2001 was $1 939 654, for 2002–2003, $2 222 654.
4   UNICEF's expenditure in 2001 was $1 246 million, of which $240 million was for immunization and $67 million for HIV/AIDS programmes: see *2002 UNICEF Annual Report*.
5   UNDP's regular resources in 2000 were $634 million. Its total expenditures in the same year were $702 million, of which 62% were entrusted to governments for national execution (UN Doc. DP/2001/22, 25 July 2001, *Annual Review of the Financial Situation, 2000*).
6   UNAIDS' annual budget is $60 million and has a staff of 129 professionals. See UNAIDS *Mission Statement*.
7   See World Bank *Annual Report 2002*.
8   For instance, Bill Gates combined business meetings with visits to AIDS clinics connected with his Foundation during his four-day tour in India in November 2002: see *International Herald Tribune (IHT)*, 12 November 2002.

PART I
THE UNITED NATIONS
AND THE WORLD HEALTH
ORGANIZATION

Chapter 1

United Nations Organizations and Business

On 31 January 1999, speaking at the World Economic Forum in Davos, Switzerland, United Nations Secretary-General Kofi Annan first proposed the Global Compact (United Nations, 2002). Amid a rising concern about the effects of globalization, he called on business leaders to join this international initiative that would bring companies together with UN agencies, labour, non-governmental organizations and other civil society actors[1] to foster action and partnerships in the pursuit of good corporate citizenship.

On 5 July 1999, Annan and International Chamber of Commerce President Adnan Kassar affirmed that the UN goals of peace and development are compatible with business goals of wealth and prosperity. Both acknowledged that the universal values promoted by the UN are the very values that can help safeguard open markets and expand the benefits of globalization (UNA of the USA, 2000).

In 1998, Annan had already engaged in a dialogue with the international business community which he called 'mutually beneficial' (United Nations, 1998). For Annan, business has a stake in the soft infrastructure produced by the UN system – the norms, standards and best practices on which the smooth flow of international transactions depends, UN work on behalf of peace, human rights and development. In turn, the UN appreciates that business has the capacity, technology and expertise necessary to fuel economic growth.

The Global Compact was officially launched at UN headquarters on 26 July 2000, in a meeting attended by senior executives from more than 50 major corporations and the leaders of a few labour, human rights and development organizations.

The concept and implementation of the Global Compact were due to the initiative and efforts of Annan, without preliminary submission to and endorsement by Member States. It raised immediate protests from a number of NGOs, as an 'unholy alliance' with profit-making enterprises which had been the target of condemnations by UN bodies and developing countries in past decades.

Engagement with the business community would parallel, and perhaps rival, the long-standing, close relationships the UN has with NGOs, its first and often indispensable partners in the fields of human rights, the environment, development, trade issues, humanitarian assistance and the issues of women and children.

The first UN partners: the NGOs

Article 71 of the UN Charter authorized the Economic and Social Council 'to make suitable arrangements for consultation with non-governmental organizations which are concerned with matters within its competence'. The Principles to be applied in establishing consultative relations between NGOs and the Council were revised in 1996.[2] They provide that the aims and purposes of the NGO must be in conformity with the spirit, purposes and principles of the UN Charter. The NGO must undertake to support the work of the UN and to promote knowledge of its principles and activities. The NGO's programme of work must be of direct relevance to the aims and purposes of the UN. The NGO must be of recognized standing within the particular field of its competence or of a representative character. The NGOs applying for consultative status may be at the national, sub-regional, regional or international levels. End 2002, there were 2143 NGOs in consultative status with the Council, and some 400 NGOs accredited to the Commission on Sustainable Development, a subsidiary body of the Council.

Large numbers of NGOs have attended large-scale international conferences on special themes, such as population, the status of women, the environment. For example, the UN Conference on the Environment and Development in Rio de Janeiro in 1992, registered 1400 NGO representatives: only a few had consultative status with the Council (Weiss & Gordenker, 1996).

Most UN agencies and funds have set up their own consultative status with NGOs. Among them, the UNESCO National Commissions and the NGO Committee on UNICEF, which have built strong bridges with professional groups, NGOs and even individual citizens. The same applies to the FAO Freedom from Hunger Campaign. The Programme Coordinating Board of the Joint UN Programme on HIV/AIDS (UNAIDS) includes five representatives of NGOs, including associations of people living with AIDS, besides government representatives.

NGOs work at both policy and operational levels. They mobilize public opinion, they act as counter-powers, lobby and challenge governments and intergovernmental bodies, they monitor and challenge business organizations. Many carry out the field work of UN agencies such as the UNHCR and UNICEF.

The UN and transnational corporations: from opposition to cooperation

In 1974 and 1975, the UN General Assembly voted for the establishment of a New International Economic Order, against the will of the industrialized countries. In this context, Transnational Corporations (TNCs) were criticized by Third World and socialist countries for their investment and commercial practices, their political pressures, and charged with corruption. They claimed that TNCs were impeding development and competing unfairly on a global basis. The new automatic majority of developing countries in UN bodies promoted the formulation of codes of conduct to regulate transactions between TNCs and host governments. In 1974, the UN established in New York an intergovernmental Commission on Transnational Corporations (UNCTC). In 1975, a newly created UN Center on TNCs began work on a code of conduct. Also in 1975, negotiations started at the United Nations Conference on Trade and Development (UNCTAD) on restrictive business practices and on the transfer of technology, but no agreement was reached on an International Code of Conduct for Transnational Corporations. Codes on specific products were however approved: in 1981, the International Code of Marketing of Breast-milk

Substitutes, sponsored by WHO and UNICEF (see Chapter 3), – in 1985, the FAO Code of Conduct on the Distribution and Use of Pesticides and in 1988 the WHO Ethical Criteria for Medicinal Drug Promotion.

The political and economic climates changed in the 1980s. TNCs were now seen as agents of the investment, trade and technology transfer required for development. Reflecting the trend towards neo-liberalism and the development of economic globalization, UN policy towards TNCs changed course (Utting, 2001). Instead of trying to regulate foreign direct investment (FDI), UN agencies like UNCTAD sought to facilitate the access of developing countries to FDI. Deregulation and privatization were encouraged. UNCTC ceased to function as a separate entity in 1992.

The UN General Assembly recognized in 1993 the importance of the market and the private sector for the efficient functioning of economies in various stages of development (A/RES/48/180). The resolution recalled with satisfaction the active collaboration between the UN system and private sector associations, such as the on-going efforts of UNDP with the International Chamber of Commerce, the Business Council for Sustainable Development and the Chamber of Commerce and Industry of the Group of 77. The Assembly encouraged organs, organizations and bodies of the UN system to foster active partnerships between public and private entities.

Another resolution adopted by the UN General Assembly in February 1998 (A/RES/52/209) recognized that business and industry, including TNCs, play a crucial role in the social and economic development of countries and recognized the need to increase private sector involvement in the provision of infrastructure services, *inter alia*, through joint ventures between public and private entities. Yet another resolution adopted in 2000 (A/RES/54/204) noted, *inter alia,* the efforts of the Secretary-General to create partnerships with the private sector. However, it did not give free rein to business: the resolution encouraged governments to create an environment enabling businesses to conduct their activities in a humane, sustainable and socially responsible way.

The climate between the public and private sectors was also changing in industrialized countries. In May 2001, Franz Schoser, then Chief Executive of the German Association of Chambers of Commerce and Industry said in a meeting with journalists: 'In the seventies, German development policy worked against the private sector. In the eighties, it ignored the private sector. And since the nineties, it has finally been working with the private sector'. Another German leader added that neither the public nor the private sectors can cope alone with the huge development challenges facing us (Rabe, 2002).

The Global Compact, a voluntary network

At the core of this network are the Global Compact Office at the UN headquarters, and four UN agencies, the International Labour Organization (ILO), the Office of the UN High Commissioner for Human Rights (UNHCHR), the UN Environmental Programme (UNEP) and the UN Development Programme (UNDP). It seeks to involve governments, companies, labour, civil society organizations and the UN as convener and facilitator.

The Compact is a voluntary corporate citizenship initiative. It is not a regulatory instrument: it does not 'police' or enforce the behaviour or actions of companies. It relies on the enlightened self-interest of companies, labour and civil society to initiate and share substantive action in pursuing the principles upon which the Compact is based. The Compact seeks to make globalization more equitable – and thus more sustainable – for the vast numbers currently excluded from the international marketplace. For the Secretary-General, the Compact is also 'a chance for the UN to renew itself from within, and to gain greater relevance in the 21st century by showing it can work with non-state actors, as well as states, to achieve the broad goals on which its members have agreed' (United Nations, 2002). It aims at filling the void between regulatory regimes, at one end of the spectrum, and voluntary codes of industry conduct, at the other.

The Compact asks companies to embrace, support and enact, within their sphere of influence, a set of core values in the areas of human rights, labour standards and the environment. The Compact's nine principles are derived from the Universal Declaration of Human Rights, the ILO Declaration on Fundamental Principles and Rights at Work, and the Rio Declaration on Environment and Development (see below, Presentation 1.1). A participating company needs to bring about positive change only in those areas that are relevant to its business operations.

Presentation 1.1

The Nine Principles of the Global Compact

Human Rights
1.   Businesses should support and respect the protection of internationally proclaimed human rights; and
2.   Make sure that they are not complicit in human rights abuses.

Labour Standards
1.   Businesses should uphold the freedom of association and the effective recognition of the right to collective bargaining;
2.   The elimination of all forms of forced and compulsory labour;
3.   The effective abolition of child labour; and
4.   Eliminate discrimination in respect of employment and occupation.

Environment
1.   Businesses should support a precautionary approach to environmental challenges;
2.   Undertake initiatives to promote greater environmental responsibility; and
3.   Encourage the development and diffusion of environmentally friendly technologies.

Source: *The Global Compact, Corporate Leadership in the World Economy* UN, January 2001.

In January 2002, the Secretary-General convened an Advisory Council on the Global Compact composed of senior business executives, international labour leaders, public policy experts, and heads of civil society organizations across the world (United Nations, 2002). Members of the Council are addressing four related priorities: 1), safeguarding the integrity of the Global Compact; 2) serving as advocates of the Compact; 3) providing expertise relating to the Compact's focus area; and 4) offering advice on policy and strategy. The Compact has initiated several Policy Dialogues which have brought together companies with labour and civil society organizations. Topics have included 'The Role of Business in Zones of Conflict', 'Business and Sustainable Development'. In the fledging Learning Forum, companies will be submitting on the Compact website annual examples of how they apply one or more of the nine principles. They will be encouraged to develop case studies. A global academic network will oversee these processes. The Compact will also encourage public-private partnerships that support UN goals. Finally, Global Compact Outreach promotes global support for the Compact at national level.

A Working Group on Company Participation and Civil Society Engagement will propose safeguards to ensure that companies engaged in Compact activities do not abuse or exploit their affiliation with the UN.

Two conditions must be met for companies to be identified as participants in the Global Compact initiative. First, companies must submit a formal letter of intent to the Secretary-General affirming their commitment to the nine principles. Secondly, the companies must submit annually an example of their efforts to uphold and implement one or more of the nine principles. If both requirements are fulfilled, a company's identity and their submitted example will be posted on the Compact website. Restrictions apply to the use of the Compact logo and to the general UN logo. No financial contributions from companies are accepted. All funding for the Compact comes from member states' donations and not-for-profit entities.

By the end of 2002, 563 companies worldwide had pledged support for the Compact and were implementing its principles.[3] Among them, large petroleum, chemical and pharmaceutical companies, international banks, telecommunication firms, car and other manufacturers. The country distribution was uneven: 82 companies in India, 91 in the Philippines, 117 in Spain, and only 35 in the USA. Companies in 18 European countries were participants, 11 from Asian countries, only five from Latin American countries and from Africa.

Why do companies join? According to Ruggie[4] (2000), a major reason is the protection and promotion of the company brand. Another reason is that some companies have come to view global corporate social responsibility as a natural extension of corporate social responsibility in their home countries, as one of the rules of the game in the new global market place. For some companies in the cutting edge industries, more elevated social purposes are becoming part of corporate culture, aimed at attracting the very best candidates for employment. Finally, there may be companies looking to the Compact for a free ride, mere publicity, a 'bluewash' instead of good practices.

Other participants included the International Chamber of Commerce,[5] the International Organization of Employers and other International Business Associations. Among several labour organizations is the International Confederation of Free Trade Unions, representing 156 million members in 221 national trade union centres from 148 countries. Among civil society organizations are Amnesty International and Human Rights Watch, the Save the Children Alliance, the World Wide Fund for Nature (WWF), Transparency International, and a number of academic institutions.

NGOs against the Global Compact

Since March 1999, CorpWatch[6] has led an international campaign to document and expose the growing number of partnerships between various UN agencies and corporations with poor human rights and environmental records. It proposed an alternative relationship between the UN and corporations, one in which the UN would serve as counterbalance to corporate-led globalization. CorpWatch is the secretariat of the Alliance for a Corporate-Free United Nations.

In September 2000, it published a report (Bruno and Karliner, 2000) on Corporate Partnerships at the United Nations, 'Tangled Up in Blue'. The report argued that corporate influence at the UN was already too great, and that new partnerships were leading down a slippery road toward the partial privatization and commercialization of the UN system itself. It stated that the Secretary-General's Office and UN agencies such as UNICEF, UNDP, WHO, and UNESCO were partnering with corporations known for human, labour and environmental rights violations. For CorpWatch, the Global Compact and its cousin partnerships at other UN agencies were threatening the mission and the integrity of the UN.

According to the report, the Global Compact had four major problems:

- Wrong companies: The Secretary-General had shown poor judgment by allowing human rights, labour and environmental violators to join;
- Wrong relationships: Clearly the UN must have interactions with corporations, as when they procure goods and services or to hold them accountable, but it should not aspire to 'partnership';
- Wrong image: The UN positive image is vulnerable to being sullied by corporate criminals, while companies get a chance to 'bluewash' their image by wrapping themselves in the flag of the UN;
- No monitoring or Enforcement: Companies that sign-up get to declare their allegiance to UN principles without making a commitment to follow them.

In 2001, CorpWatch said that many of the signatories to the Compact had violated some of the nine principles and blamed UNDP, UNESCO, the UNHCR and WHO for their partnership or association with corporations known for such violations (CorpWatch, 2001).

In a letter to Kofi Annan dated 29 January 2002, the Alliance for a Corporate-Free UN wrote that they agreed with the Secretary-General's motivation that the Compact is to improve corporate behaviour. However, they believe that the Compact, as currently designed, has serious flaws that threaten the integrity and mission of the UN. They believe that the Compact allows companies to improve their reputation through association with the UN, without committing to concrete changes in corporate behaviour. It allows these corporations, and the private sector as a whole, to block substantial measures for sustainability and accountability, even to oppose agreements under the framework of the UN itself, while offering only token changes when convenient. The letter then attached documentation of alleged violations by Aventis, Nike, Unilever, Norsk Hydro, Rio Tinto and the International Chamber of Commerce. It then proposed to redesign the Compact as the Global Accountability Compact. This would not be an equal partnership between sectors that do not share all values and goals. The new Compact companies must agree to support the entry into force and implementation of multilateral agreements under UN auspices. The Compact's nine principles should be further defined so as to be able to determine whether companies are implementing them or not. A forum should be established to which citizens and NGOs could bring evidence of violations of the principles by Compact companies. The complanies could bring their own evidence. The UN would determine whether a violation had occurred, and if so, present the company with a timetable for correcting the violation in order to avoid suspension from the Compact.

Paul Hawken, founder of the Sausalito-based Natural Capital Institute (Go-Between, 2002) wrote in 2002:

> There is a growing worldwide movement towards corporate responsibility and sustainability, led in many cases by companies whose history and products have brought damage and suffering to the world ... Transnational corporations ... have prevented the strengthening of environmental and labour laws and they have led the effort to eliminate the ability of smaller, more vulnerable nations to determine their own economic destiny. In other words, they embrace 'sustainability' as long as they can make money and it doesn't change their overall purpose , which is to grow faster than the overall world economy and population and increase their share of the world's economic output to the benefit of a small number of shareholders.

Ruggie (2000) has replied in part to these criticisms. In short, the Global Compact is not a Code of Conduct. Its aim is to engage the relevant social actors in a learning experience based on identifying and promoting good practices. Should some corporate participants in the Compact be disqualified because of their past actions? It makes no sense for the UN to engage only companies that are already perfect. Companies are asked for a genuine commitment to work with the UN: if the UN has any doubt about the sincerity of that commitment, the company is not invited to join the Compact. The hope and expectation is that good practices will help drive out bad ones through the power of dialogue, transparency, advocacy and competition. The use of the UN logo is strictly controlled by the UN Office of Legal Affairs on a case-by-case basis. No authorization is given for commercial purposes. Contrary to a few NGOs, the Global Compact does not reject the phenomenon of globalization itself. Rejectionism will not solve poverty. A globalization embedded in universal values and principles, better managed by 'good governance' at both national and international levels, may help in solving some of the problems.

Ruggie added (2001): The Compact is 'a network of autonomous actors, each with different interests and needs that intersect only partially'. This was both the chief weakness and the main strength of the Compact.

However, the financial scandals of late 2001 and 2002 (Enron, WorldCom and others) have given new arguments to the promoters of a 'Corporate-free UN', or, at least to those who wish the UN to exercise great caution in its relations with the private sector.

The risks entailed in close UN/business relations were revealed in the Report of the UN Secretary-General on the work of the Organization for 1999 (Doc. A/54/1, paragraphs 341 and 342). Following reports of the illegal export and improper retention of intellectual property by those associated with a UN project, the Investigation Section of the Office of Internal Oversight Services (OIOS) examined UN/private sector partnerships involving electronic commerce. The investigation uncovered extensive solicitations of funds and unauthorized commercial agreements between UN staff and private individuals and companies. It also uncovered private sector interests in a UN-sponsored programme providing technical assistance to economically disadvantaged countries. OIOS made recommendations to remedy these abuses and for tighter controls on partnerships with the private sector. OIOS has recommended that the UN enforce high ethical and legal standards in its commercial dealings with outside entities. In the view of the Joint Inspection Unit, this case highlighted the crucial importance attached to the use of the UN name by private sector technology firms, and the significant profits which could derive from it (JIU, 1999, 16).

The relations of UN organizations with business

Relations of UN organizations with business are not new: They predate the creation of the Global Compact and now run in parallel with it (JIU, 1999). They have not raised the same controversies and accusations as the Compact.

The UN procurement requirements have created extensive commercial links with the private sector. Overall, the UN represents an annual market of $3 billion for supplies of virtually all types of goods and services. The value of business opportunities provided by the UN system and the Developing Banks is estimated at $30 billion annually.

The private sector has long participated in the normative and standard-setting work of the UN. Even prior to the creation of the UN, the predecessors of the World Intellectual Property Organization, and then the Organization, have worked closely with representatives of the private sector for over a century, in developing norms in its field. Created in 1919, the International Labour Organisation, due to its unique tripartite structure, includes private employers' and workers' representatives together with governments in the formulation and approval of labour Conventions, and in its technical cooperation programmes. The business community has been closely involved in the work of the Economic Commission for Europe for the standardization of trade documents. Oil, chemical and shipping industries contribute significantly to the regulatory work of the International Maritime Organization. FAO has also a long history of cooperation with the private sector in regulatory and normative programmes such as the Codex Alimentarius of FAO and WHO.

UNICEF has the most extensive corporate involvement of any single UN agency, but exercises 'due diligence' in selecting business partners. For instance, Warner

Brothers, Turner Network Television, Time for Kids and Coinstar support the Trick or Trade UNICEF campaign. British Airways, the Sheraton and Westin hotel chains and American Express are involved in UNICEF marketing efforts linked to specific fund-raising activities. However, UNICEF attaches ethical strings to its supply contracts, favouring companies that avoid links with such activities as landmine production and exploitative child labour. The agency does not deal with cigarette companies or accept contributions from manufacturers of infant formula (UNICEF, 1999).

WHO's recent opening to business, the creation of several international public/ private partnerships for health, are reviewed in the remaining parts of this book.

Conclusion

As noted by Nelson (2002), in today's world, achieving global objectives, such as peace and security, development and poverty eradication, environmental protection, human rights, democracy and good governance, is critical not only to the UN's agenda but also to long-term business success and survival.

Following the Millennium Declaration, adopted on 8 September 2000 by world leaders, the UN General Assembly took note in 2001 of the Millennium Development Goals defined by UN bodies, the World Bank, the International Monetary Fund and the Organization for Economic Cooperation and Development. The eight goals to be achieved by 2015 are:

- halving extreme poverty and hunger;
- achieving universal primary education;
- promoting gender equality;
- reducing under-five mortality by two-thirds;
- reducing maternal mortality by three-quarters;
- reversing the spread of HIV/AIDS, tuberculosis and malaria;
- ensuring environmental sustainability;
- developing a global partnership for development, with targets for aid, trade and debt relief.

Working with governments, other intergovernmental organizations and NGOs, with uneven success, and faced with these ambitious goals, the UN has recently called publicly on the private sector for help. One reason was to obtain additional funds in times of reduced public aid. Public funds for development, worldwide, have been estimated at around $50 billion for roughly ten years. In contrast, over the same period of time, private investments into developing countries have been growing steadily, coming close to $200 billion per annum in the late 1990s (Rabe, 2002). Where private companies invest, analysts argue that they create jobs and new sources of income, train local staff and transfer new technologies to partner countries. Hence, the UN's motivation in joining forces with business and cooperate in those areas where public and private interests might overlap.

A broader reason is to extend UN's influence in making economic globalization sustainable and more equitable, by adding business, its dominant engine, to its institutional partners, the governments, and its traditional partners, the NGOs.

Another reason, internal to the organization itself, is to benefit from business dynamism, adaptability and technology offered by the private sector. In his plans for UN reform, Kofi Annan expected that the new relationship with business would provoke a new entrepreneur-type spirit in the UN bureaucracy.

The expected benefits for the UN are clear. The potential benefits for business are less evident.

The basic objective of business firms is to make profit in order to satisfy their shareholders. Preventing war and maintaining peace, fighting world poverty, promoting gender equality or fighting epidemics is a responsibility of governments and IGOs, with the voluntary support of NGOs, but not of business. Business firms are accountable to their shareholders, to national governments – they must respect national laws – they must satisfy their customers, their well-understood interest is to have satisfied and productive employees, but any other, broader goal can only be an optional luxury to those basic obligations. Large transnational corporations and business-issued foundations benefit from their participation in joint public-private partnerships in specific areas, allocating relatively small financial contributions and efforts to specific visible schemes. Their reputation is then enhanced by their participation with prestigious UN organizations in worthy projects.

Except for a number of progressive enterprises, the main motivation of many in joining the Global Compact and public/private partnerships may be to enhance their reputation and relations with various stakeholders, and promote their image among customers conscious of development issues in rich countries, and among governments and populations in poor countries, where assistance by UN bodies is known and appreciated. It may be a response to NGO criticisms of firms' violations of international conventions and standards in the fields of human rights, labour law and the environment.

As noted by Hamm (2002), the Pact's non-binding character, generality and diffuseness could appear to companies as a welcome alternative to tougher national or international legislation and codes of conduct. Unlike binding instruments and codes, the Pact can deliver a corporate identification effect simply by means of symbols (the UN and its logo) and thus serve the companies' marketing interests. Adhering to the voluntary Pact would in fact stave off binding national and international regulation.

Critics charge that the Compact's main ill-advised effect is to legitimize big business and to welcome companies with tarnished reputations. In 1999, NGOs have criticized the involvement of the Compact, of the UNHCR and of the International Committee of the Red Cross in the Business Humanitarian Forum, with Unocal Corporation, an oil company, the United Technologies Corporation, a military contractor, Nestlé, Rio Tinto, a mining conglomerate and others, all targets of NGO campaigns. Also in 1999, UNDP had to halt the creation of the Global Sustainable Development Facility following NGO opposition to the proposed financial participation of global corporations with tarnished records on human rights, labour and the environment. Ruggie's reply that the Compact cannot only engage with 'perfect' companies is not tenable, unless the behaviour of 'imperfect' companies joining the Compact is carefully monitored.

The UN opening to business: setting limits

Carol Bellamy, the UNICEF Executive Director, said it plainly: 'It is dangerous to assume that the goals of the private sector are somehow synonymous with those of the UN, because they most emphatically are not ... In coming together with the private sector, the UN must carefully, and constantly, appraise the relationship ... the heart of the matter is the exercise of "due diligence"' (UNICEF, 1999).

Has Kofi Annan exerted 'due diligence' in launching the Compact as a voluntary, non-binding, non-assessing network? Is there a useful place for the Compact between regulatory regimes and voluntary codes? Is voluntarism by business firms, dialogue between the UN and the private sector and sharing of best practices an effective project?

The Compact needs improvement. The main concerns are related to selection criteria, disclosure and monitoring. There is a need for clearer criteria for the admission of enterprises. The behaviour of these enterprises, following admission, should be monitored and evaluated by an independent group[7] on the basis of set criteria, and not only by NGOs. There should be clear guidelines on targets which have been met within a certain timeframe. The participation of companies failing standards should be stopped.

In 2002, the Compact joined forces with the Global Reporting Initiative (GRI)(Go Between, 2002). The Initiative was established in 1997 by the US-based Coalition for Environmentally Responsible Economies (CERES) in collaboration with UNEP: It was formally inaugurated on 4 April 2002 at UN headquarters in New York. An international sustainability reporting institution, its mandate is to develop globally applicable guidelines for reporting on economic, environmental, and social performance. GRI will start communicating directly with all companies participating with the Compact. The collaboration GRI-Compact should increase the transparency of reports submitted by companies, and therefore assist in the evaluation of their performance and adhesion to the Compact's nine principles.

A certain lack of transparency in the development of the Global Compact is apparent, insofar as the 'opposition' is not invited to comment. NGOs fair or unfair criticisms should be openly ventilated and publicized on the Compact website. The UN should not fear confrontation: alleged shortcomings of specific companies should be made public, leading to rebuttals, discussions and evaluations. The first report on the Global Compact's Progress and Activities (UN, 2002) reports only on achievements and plans. It refers to 'daunting challenges' which are not identified. The participation of civil society, including trade unions, academics and NGOs, is not given due credit: the problems raised by these 'other' partners, such as conflicts of interests, self-censorship, the poor choice of some partners, the risks to UN independence and credibility, are not mentioned, nor the response of the Compact Office to these problems. There is a need for a counterweight to business' own weight and influence.

The UN agencies should develop guidelines for working with the business community and for setting up partnerships involving business firms and business-issued foundations.

Finally, UN organizations should not exclude the development of binding international conventions, such as the Framework Convention on Tobacco Control, or Codes, such as the International Code of Marketing of Breast-Milk Substitutes, in supplement to voluntary initiatives such as the Global Compact. They are aware that such development will face the opposition of the USA and other rich countries, and of the transnational corporations. Heads of UN secretariats will therefore need courage and determination in initiating such schemes.

Is the Global Compact a success or a failure? It is too early to pass a judgment. On the positive side, it has opened the UN system to the business world, a world which was earlier rejected *en bloc* on ideological terms, or criticized, or now, excessively eulogized or feared. UN/private partnerships are playing a useful role in tackling specific technical problems, with a broader visibility than if they were only carried out by UN bodies. On the negative side, the name and integrity of the UN remains in danger of being abused by its association with business firms whose goals are different, if not in opposition with those of the Organization.

There is therefore a need for strengthening the position of the UN organizations vs. business and allowing for a healthy participation of civil society organizations.

At the same time, in spite of its lofty objectives, it should be realized that initiatives such as the Global Compact are only a 'drop in the ocean' in the words of Hamm (2002). Ruggie (2001) has himself recognized that 'anyone who sees in the Global Compact the cure for globalization's many ills does not sufficiently grasp the fragile basis of all such networks'.

There are other multi-stakeholders alliances, such as the Global Environmental Facility, the Commission on Sustainable Development, the UN Fund for International Partnerships, Business Partners for Development, and many partnerships joining UN bodies with governments, foundations, business and NGOs. Neither the Compact nor those alliances will, on their own, make globalization more equitable for all populations, they will not reduce world-wide poverty. While the Compact will help in making a number of companies more aware of international standards in human rights, labour laws and the environment, there is no guarantee that business firms will change their colours. While public/private partnerships are useful innovative ventures to achieve limited, well-defined objectives, they will not solve the fundamentals of unsustainable development and social injustice (Utting, 2002). These include major political, economic, social and cultural issues. Among others, poor governance, civil wars, epidemics, gross imbalances in power relations between groups and nations, weak states, North-South trade and debt.

Notes

1   Civil Society organizations have been defined as movements, entities, institutions autonomous from the state which in principle, are non-profit-making, act locally, nationally and internationally, in defence and promotion of social, economic and cultural interests and for mutual benefit. They include professional associations, cooperatives,

village development communities, indigenous peoples, women and youth groups, networks for homework, religious and cultural associations, academic institutions, media centers and intellectual and research entities (JIU, 2002).

2   ECOSOC Resolution 1996/31, revising Resolution 1296 (XLIV) of 1968.

3   There are 65,000 transnational corporations in the world.

4   From 1997 to 2001, John G. Ruggie was Assistant Secretary-General and chief adviser for strategic planning to the UN Secretary-General. He was the main inspirer of the Global Compact. He is now Kirkpatrick Professor of International Affairs at Harvard University's School of Government and faculty associate of its Center for Business and Government.

5   The International Chamber of Commerce and the US Chamber of Commerce had urged ratification of the UN Charter in 1945 (Tesner, 2000, xx).

6   CorpWatch was formerly known as the Transnational Resource & Action Center (TRAC).

7   The group could include representatives from IGOs, governments, TNCs, NGOs, experts and academics.

Chapter 2

The World Health Organization and Business

Kofi Annan launched the UN Global Compact in July 2000. In May 1998, Dr Gro Harlem Brundtland, who had been elected by the World Health Assembly on 13 May, said: 'We must reach out to the private sector ... We need open and constructive relations with the private sector and industry, knowing where our roles differ and where they may complement each other. I invite industry to join in a dialogue on the key issues facing us' (WHO, 1998a).[1]

In a report issued in December 2001, the Commission on Macroeconomics and Health, established by WHO, showed that investing in health in developing countries saves lives and produces clear and measurable financial returns. According to the Commission, the well-targeted spending of $66 billion a year by 2015 could save as many as eight million lives a year and generate six-fold economic benefits, more than $360 billion a year by 2020. For Dr Brundtland, this is not a battle that can be won by international organizations and governments alone: it is a global challenge to individuals, companies and organizations in every country. It opened, for WHO and for countries, a new era of public-private partnerships (WHO, 2002a).

Past and present relations with business

WHO relations with business did not start with Dr Brundtland. The first partnership between WHO, scientists and vaccine manufacturers, the influenza network, was launched in 1948, at the creation of WHO. It now links 110 National Influenza Centers in 83 countries, and four WHO Collaborating Centers for Virus Reference and Research in Atlanta, London, Melbourne and Tokyo.

Over the years, WHO Programmes have had direct or indirect contacts with industry in such areas as malaria control or eradication (insecticides), water supplies, smallpox eradication (vaccination devices and vaccines), research and training in tropical diseases (malaria, leprosy, onchocerciasis), essential drugs, HIV/ AIDS prevention and control. While most of the supplies needed for operational programmes were generally provided by UNICEF, UNDP, the World Bank, UNFPA and others, WHO maintained a small but not insignificant programme of purchases of supplies and equipment.[2]

In 1988, a major partnership was established with other UN agencies, the World Bank, governments and NGOs. Merck & Co donated ivermectin for large-scale treatment of river blindness (see Chapter 6). Also in 1988, the Global Poliomyelitis Eradication Programme was launched by WHO (see Chapter 7). It included among its many partners, UNICEF, the US Centers for Disease Control and Prevention, governments and several foundations, Rotary International, the Gates Foundation and the UN Foundation. During the 1990s, vaccine and pharmaceuticals manufacturers collaborated with donor agencies and scientists in many countries, under the leadership of WHO, to carry out research aimed at improving the treatment of sleeping sickness, leprosy, malaria and human fascioliasis. In 1996, WHO was one of the six co-sponsors of the Joint UN Programme on HIV/AIDS (UNAIDS), together with UNICEF, UNDP, UNFPA, UNESCO and the World Bank (Chapter 5). UNAIDS collaborates with The Prince of Wales Business Leaders Forum, Rotary International, the Conference Board (comprised of senior executives from all industries), the World Economic Forum. In 1997, partnerships were created to combat meningitis and rabies.

Initiated in 1998, the Global Alliance to Eliminate Lymphatic Filariasis was officially formed in May 2000. In addition to National Ministries of Health, the World Bank, UNICEF and WHO, international development agencies, NGOs, academia and research institutions, it includes three industry partners, Binax, Inc., Merck & Co., Inc. and GlaxoSmithKline (WHO, 1999a). One of the key projects initiated by Dr Brundtland, Roll-Back Malaria, a new campaign to fight malaria was launched in 1998 by UNICEF, the World Bank and WHO (Chapter 8). It also includes national governments, development agencies and banks, the private sector and the media. In 1999, WHO, the World Bank, a few governments and foundations, the International Federation of Pharmaceutical Manufacturers Associations (IFPMA) and other private sector enterprises joined together to create the Medicines for Malaria Venture. The Global Alliance for Vaccines and Immunization (GAVI) was created in January 2000 (Chapter 9). It includes UNICEF, WHO, the World Bank, foundations and IFPMA.

WHO has worked with the Association of Oil and Gas Producers to help establish strategic health management principles and guidelines for this industry. Another new venture is WHO's cooperation agreement with the World Alliance for Community Health, a not-for-profit organization set up by five international mining companies (WHO, 1999b).

WHO maintains close collaboration with a number of business-issued, or business-related, foundations. Among them, the Nippon Foundation (leprosy), Rotary International (polio), Eli Lilly (mental health), Lions Club International (blindness), the Rockefeller Foundation (vaccines, tropical disease research, and others), the David and Lucille Packard Foundation (reproductive health) and the Hewlett Foundation (human reproduction). A major development has been the creation of the United Nations Foundation, Inc. early 1998 and the endowment of $17 thousand million made by the Bill and Melinda Gates Foundation.

In summary, WHO collaborates with a number of private sector firms: among them, Merck & Co. (onchocerciasis), GlaxoSmithKline (lymphatic filiarisis, malaria), the Novartis Group (malaria, leprosy), Pasteur Mérieux Connaught (polio). It collaborates with IFPMA and various industry groups. Several of its programmes are supported by business-related foundations.

NGOs' protests

A few influential NGOs in official relations with WHO have raised objections or concerns about WHO's 'increasing enthusiasm' for public/private interaction. Seeing this process as unstoppable, they made proposals to protect WHO's good name against potential excessive influence from business.

Health Action International (HAI) saw an inherent conflict between commercial and public health goals. WHO, as the primary public health body in the world, must ensure that public health interests are paramount. The organization must perform its functions independently from commercial influence.[3] In a statement submitted on 22 January 2001 to the 107th Executive Board Meeting, Consumers International, HAI and the International Baby Food Action Network (IBFAN) raised the following concerns: – do public-private interactions contribute to equity in health care? – do they encourage vertical programmes focused on diseases calling for high technologically expensive solutions rather than those identified as national public health priorities? – are they a quick fix or do they contribute to sustainable health benefits? – are these well-publicized collaborations actually about donor image-building, product development and marketing?

World Vision had strong reservations about WHO's interaction with commercial enterprises. It saw a real danger in this collaboration. It was opposed to trading ethical values for short term gain for WHO. The NGO had seen how the industries manipulate and interpret any guidelines to their advantage. It was against the secondment of staff from TNCs to WHO.[4]

While Save the Children did not see joint initiatives between WHO and the commercial sector as the most effective or desirable path for WHO, it accepted that in certain strongly safeguarded circumstances, they may be necessary. The NGO then offered suggestions: Proposals for public-private interactions should contain not only a clear statement of purpose, but specific outcomes with defined benefits to the health of specific groups, and indicators to evaluate those. Guidelines for staff on handling public-private interactions specific to commodity donations and lower prices for commodities should incorporate principles of good practice based on critical research and a transparent consultative process with relevant stakeholders. Guidelines on conflict of interest should emphasize the need for transparency in documenting the nature and interests of all relevant parties. In order to achieve a behaviour change among companies that had a negative impact on health, WHO should consult relevant civil society organizations. WHO should establish a mechanism for public hearings in relation to WHO's work themes that examined good and bad practices regarding companies' impact on health. The tool being developed to assess the good standing of companies with whom interaction was envisaged should be independent and sufficiently robust to serve as an incentive to companies to improve their standards of practice. The evaluation of the impact of public-private interactions on the independence of WHO should be carried out externally (WHO, 2002a).

Incidents and problems

It is not in the interest of WHO to admit publicly that it has experienced problems in its interaction with business. Business firms would rather praise their cooperation and generosity towards WHO rather than expose less admirable examples of abusive influence or even corruption on either side. Such problems are therefore rarely made public. The following examples show they have existed before 1998 as well as after 1998, when WHO's interaction with business was openly promoted and expanded.

Before 1998

At the national level, tobacco companies have long applied a calculated and well-financed strategy to deflect attention from the consequences of smoking on health and to prevent appropriate legislation. At the international level, its influence within WHO over many years has only been revealed publicly in a WHO report issued in 2000 (WHO, 2000). The report said that tobacco companies 'sought to divert attention from the public health issues raised by tobacco use, to reduce budgets for the scientific and policy activities carried out by WHO, to pit other UN agencies against WHO, to convince developing countries that WHO's tobacco control programme was a "first world" agenda carried out at the expense of the developing world, to distort the results of important scientific studies on tobacco and to discredit WHO as an institution' (see Chapter 10).

Among more limited incidents, during the May 1987 session of the WHO Executive Board, two Board members referred to the distribution of material by a NGO in official relations with WHO which had been handed to the delegations directly. They considered this material as inappropriate commercial advertising, provocative, not in the best taste and an abuse of their official relations status. In an unsatisfactory reply which seemed to expose the danger of a close relation with a business-related NGO, this NGO replied later that the document had been issued in the context of a WHO technical meeting on food safety to which they had been invited and had sent two delegates. Assuring the Board members of its good faith, the document was to illustrate the way the NGO was fulfilling its responsibilities (WHO, 1987).

In January 1990, the International Organization of Consumers' Unions (IOCU) informed the WHO Standing Committee on Non-governmental Organizations that views expressed in a restricted document reviewed by the Committee in January 1989 had been improperly used by 'outside interests' (WHO, 1990). The Director-General took undisclosed 'appropriate action' in this connection.

A serious individual case of a WHO staff member conducting private business while employed by the Organization and using his position for his personal financial advantage was brought to light in a judgment of the Administrative Tribunal of the International Labour Organisation.[5] Employed as a Technical Officer in the WHO Action Programme on Essential Drugs (DAP) since 1986, G.M.'s duties included frequent travel to Africa and other countries. His contract ended on 31 October 1992. The reason for the non-renewal of his appointment was misconduct and unfitness for international public service. The organization charged that he had disregarded WHO's policy on drugs and WHO Staff Regulations: as a result, the government of Kenya had declared him *persona non grata*. He had tried to get $10,000 in commission from the International Dispensary Association (IDA), a private Dutch foundation, in exchange for a promise to persuade the Zambian government to award the Association a contract for the supply of drug kits. He solicited a 10 percent commission from a drug company in Zimbabwe in return for a promise to secure an order from the DAP. He did private consultancy work during his WHO employment. He served a firm called Misereor in recruiting and coordinating the work of other consultants and helped to produce a report for a drug distribution company, Chanpharm. The Tribunal was 'satisfied on the evidence that the WHO's reasons for not renewing his appointment might have warranted disciplinary proceedings'. The organization had the right to refuse the renewal of the fixed-term appointment for reasons that include misconduct and unsatisfactory performance.

While this case does not directly address problems of interaction between WHO and business, it shows the risks taken by the organization when business-oriented staff members lacking professional and ethical restraints use their position for personal gain and bring the organization into disrepute. Clear rules of conduct, stricter monitoring and control by the organization are needed.

After 1998

A few cases have emerged, from both internal and external sources to WHO. One clear example of an abusive practice by a commercial firm, unchecked by WHO, occurred during a WHO meeting held in 1999. A *Briefing Document for Heinz, WHO Cancer Programme* gave rather frank indications as to the benefits expected by Heinz from its sponsorship of WHO activities. Excerpts:

Sponsorship opportunities for Heinz
Enhanced global reputation for brands, particularly tomato ketchup.
Scientific and healthy living endorsement from WHO ("naughty, but nice").
Removal of trade barriers into difficult markets for Heinz products, eg China, by riding on the back of WHO health campaigns with consumers working with national governments.

Differentiation for Heinz Brands
Differentiation in the market with consumers through use of on-pack unique WHO logo (the "gold standard").

Administrative convenience of WHO sponsorship opportunity
WHO will speak the language of the sponsor and its advisers in seeking suitable ways of exploitation and promotion of the sponsorship.

Positive impact on bottom line
Grow market share by getting consumers to switch brands.
Reduce advertizing expenditure by more effective and targeted use of the WHO sponsorship in conjunction with PR on a global basis.

When informed of this commercial scenario, allowed by WHO staff unaware of business tactics, there is no doubt that WHO higher authorities put a stop to this unhealthy association. In particular, WHO would not have allowed its logo to be used for commercial purposes. It however illustrates crudely the risks of an excessively close, uncontrolled, interaction of untrained, possibly naïve WHO staff members with business representatives.

The 1999 guidelines for the management of hypertension elaborated by WHO and the International Society of Hypertension (ISH) were criticized by reputable medical journals.[6] *Prescrire* alleged that several recommendations markedly conflicted with reliable published data and questioned whether sound, independent assessment was conceivable when working parties are mainly composed of experts working more or less closely for the pharmaceutical industry. *The Lancet* referred to an open letter to the Director-General of WHO sent early 1999 by a distinguished international group of physicians claiming that 'the new [WHO-ISH] recommendations will be used to encourage an increased use of anti-hypertensive drugs, at great expense, and for little benefit ... in this particular recommendation we are left with an impression that WHO has failed its responsibility'. At its General Assembly held on 16 September 1999, members of the International Society of Drug Bulletins (ISDB) expressed concern about the 'questionable involvement of pharmaceutical companies in the compilation of WHO guidelines'. They found the guidelines on the management of hypertension 'commercially biased'. The following motion was unanimously adopted by the Assembly:

> Towards a World Health Organization independent of the pharmaceutical industry ISDB adopts the aim of engaging in actions that ensure that WHO is independent of the pharmaceutical industry, in its organization, policy decisions and funding.[7]

WHO's acceptance of Sw.Frs 10 million from Ciba Geigy for anti-diarrhoeal research was criticized by NGOs. Among others, Health Action International (HAI) had mounted a campaign attacking the use of anti-diarrhoeal products containing clioquinol, a substance which led to large-scale nerve disorders in Japan. It brought an agreement by Ciba Geigy to withdraw its clioquinol products (Chetley, 1986).

A Seminar on the Ethical Review of Clinical Research in Asian Countries was held in Thailand from 2 to 4 August 1999. It was jointly funded by SmithKline Beecham Biologicals (SKB), Belgium and the WHO Special Programme for Training and Research in Tropical Diseases (TDR), and locally organized by the Ministry of Public Health, Thailand. Other participants, including many working in regulatory agencies which have an ethical obligation of independence from business firms, were embarrassed by the participation of three SKB representatives in the meetings. The participation of only one pharmaceutical company, instead of two or more, or even better, by an industry association, was *post facto* criticized internally, as a breach of WHO's long-standing practice on commercial sponsorship.

On 12 April 1999, a Merck & Co employee joined the WHO Tobacco Free Initiative on a one-year secondment. She had previously headed the Norwegian Association of Pharmaceutical Manufacturers. In a mail distributed to all Merck employees, its Chief Executive hailed this secondment as a pioneering arrangement reflecting the new willingness of the WHO Director-General, Dr Brundtland, to form productive partnerships with the private sector. The secondment presented a 'marvelous opportunity to build bridges among Merck, the pharmaceutical industry and the global health community'. The seconded person would be an 'effective ambassador'.

Objections to this ambiguous arrangement were voiced by Consumers International, and Health Action International greeted this news with alarm. Dr Brundtland replied in June 1999 that she did not 'wish to rule out the possibility of secondments to WHO' from pharmaceutical companies'.[8] She wrote:

> In the case of the secondment to the Tobacco Free Initiative, the company had no interest in the area of smoking cessation, the person seconded brings to the project a specific and needed expertise for a time limited period, and the person is specifically excluded from involvement in activities in which the company from which she is on secondment could have any interest. Finally, there are clear undertakings on confidentiality, and on the person involved not seeking or accepting instructions from anyone outside WHO, specifically the company from which she is on secondment.

Whatever the value of WHO's arguments, questions remain. As an 'ambassador' from a pharmaceutical industry, could the seconded employee act as a loyal WHO staff member, fighting against big tobacco firms during this short period, then returning to her former functions? Why would a pharmaceutical company agree to pay for an employee to work for WHO if it thought it had nothing to gain from the arrangement? If a specific expertise was needed, could it not be obtained without risk by the appointment of an independent expert, free of any commercial interests, for a short period?

A somewhat similar situation occurred in 1996, when the World Bank established a joint two-year Fellowship with the IFPMA. The IFPMA-World Bank fellow was open to 'suitably qualified individuals presently employed in a pharmaceutical company in membership of an IFPMA Member Association'. For the duration of the fellowship, the individual would be on secondment from his/her company.

In a letter dated 19 June 1996, HAI voiced its concern about the possibility of a conflict of interest between the World Bank's commitment to promoting policies based on the WHO Essential Drugs Concept and the commercial interests of IFPMA members. HAI hoped that the World Bank's position would be reconsidered. The Associate Director of the Boston University School raised his own objections to the Fellowship. More bluntly, he wrote that there was a fundamental contradiction between the goals of IFPMA and the World Bank. The IFPMA aims to increase the consumption of patent protected pharmaceuticals at the expense of generic equivalents. The Bank's goal is to assist countries to make effective pharmaceuticals available in the most cost-effective manner.

The Bank reassured the critics that it welcomed a closer working relationship with academics, NGOs, WHO and others. The Bank did not regard the IFPMA as the sole representative of the entire pharmaceutical industry and would welcome strengthened relations with other parts of the industry and with NGOs working in this field. Bank's procurement is overwhelmingly for generics that are on the particular national essential drugs list. More specifically, the Bank representative added that the selected person would be appointed to the Bank staff during his/her tenure, and would be subject to the Bank's Principles of Staff Employment, including their requirements on the avoidance of conflicts of interest.

The Bank's policy positions will not shift because of one particular external partnership. They will shift or not in the light of international consensus, best practice and the evidence of research.[9]

The long-term association of WHO and ITC directed to the development and operation of the commercial enterprise, Market News Service for Pharmaceutical Starting Material (MNS), has been criticized by members of a WHO Expert Committee in 1994, by industrial pharmacists and by a former WHO official in 202 (Dunne, 2002). MNS provides price lists of those materials to developing countries, but apparently without verifying their origin or their quality. A 1998 report from the International Pharmaceutical Federation (FIP) said that MNS promotes the business of selected brokers, of whom only two affirmed that assured the quality of their wares. The name and logo of WHO on MNS lists may erroneously lead developing countries to believe, notwithstanding a comprehensive disclaimer, that WHO vouches for the quality of these materials. There is no evidence that WHO has taken action to remedy this situation, potentially damaging to patients and to WHO itself.

The need for ethical guidelines

WHO's wide opening to business initiated since 1998 has increased the risks of conflicts of interest between the organization and its staff, and its business partners, and the risk of damage to WHO's institutional integrity and independence, prestige and moral leadership. Hence the need to define clear ethical guidelines to be followed by the Organization and its staff in the organization's interaction with commercial enterprises.

Preventing conflicts of interest

In a report commissioned by WHO issued in June 2001, Dr Eloy Anello (Bolivia) has identified two basic categories of conflict of interest pertinent to WHO (Anello, 2001).

First, the organizational category, when a WHO programme or staff member, through their actions, creates a situation in which WHO's interaction with a commercial enterprise allows the interests of that enterprise to prevail over WHO's public health mission and objectives, although the staff member would not gain any personal benefit.

Examples: dependence on a vendor in the procurement of products, – a donation of products by a commercial enterprise, accepted and distributed by WHO: WHO may then be perceived as the marketing agent of that enterprise, – donation of funds through foundations having ties with the industry may seek to influence WHO's normative work, – earmarked donations for specific programmes may draw WHO away from priority issues, – industry members may directly or indirectly influence the formulation of treatment guidelines (see the hypertension case, above), – more generally, the attendance of industry personnel in WHO meetings and the co-sponsoring of meetings may create situations of conflicts of interest.

The second category is that of personal interest: a conflict of interest arises when a WHO staff member, in his/her relations and interactions with a commercial enterprise uses his/her professional position to influence WHO's decisions and activities in ways that could lead directly or indirectly to financial gain and/or other benefits for the staff member or family to the detriment of WHO, its reputation and interests. This definition should also include a staff member's improper use or attempt to make use of his/her official position, in relation with commercial enterprises, for his personal advantage (see the G.M. case above).

Examples: promoting the use of a product of which he/she is the owner, – accepting gifts and other favours from a commercial enterprise, – using WHO's resources for the benefit of a commercial enterprise, – shortly after leaving WHO, accepting a position with a commercial enterprise with which he/she had formal relations, such as regulatory functions, during his WHO employment.

Anello then proposed a set of principles providing a framework for managing WHO's interactions with commercial enterprises. Among them:

– mission congruence between WHO's mission and objectives and the commercial enterprise, leading to public health gains;
– selective association: WHO should avoid association with disreputable commercial enterprises;
– non-exploitation: WHO's name and logo should not be subject to exploitation by a commercial enterprise;
– the integrity and independence of WHO's normative functions should be rigorously protected from unwarranted and unethical influence by a commercial enterprise;
– a commercial enterprise in interaction with WHO should not be given a privileged competitive advantage or a monopoly;
– all interactions and agreements between WHO and a commercial enterprise should be transparent and open for disclosure and public scrutiny.

The report recommended that these principles should be defined and communicated to the WHO staff, procedures, a reference manual and a training package should be designed and applied. As a more basic requirement, a Corporate Assessment Instrument should be designed to assess and define the acceptable and appropriate levels of interaction that WHO may engage with specific commercial enterprises.

Disclosure of financial interests

In the first meeting of her Cabinet on 21 July 1998, the newly elected Director-General, Dr Brundtland announced a new policy of financial disclosure for high-level WHO officials, together with their spouses and dependent children (WHO, 1998b). They are required to submit in confidence to the Legal Counsel an annual declaration disclosing all their financial interests in the private sector, such as shareholdings or bond holdings, any patent interests, paid or unpaid directorships (paid remuneration being excluded under the present rules). The Legal Counsel then advises the Director-General on whether any holding or interest could give rise to a real or perceived conflict of interest and whether there should be a divestment, placement in trust or other administrative arrangement made with respect to such holdings and interests. As from 2000, experts engaged by the Organization or serving on expert groups and committees have been required to disclose information on financial and other interests with commercial entities, in an attempt to ensure that the best possible assessment of scientific evidence is achieved in an atmosphere free from direct or indirect pressure. In 2001, the Director-General amended Staff Rule 110.7 to require that 'a staff member who has, or whose spouse or dependent children have, any interest in (including association with) any entity with which the staff member may be required, directly or indirectly, to have official dealings on behalf of the Organization, or which has a commercial interest in the work of WHO, or a common area of activity with WHO, shall report the interest to the Director-General' (WHO, 2001b).

Institutional guidelines

In 1999, WHO released draft guidelines on working with the private sector for comment by Member States, NGOs and academia. A formal document, 'Guidelines on interaction with commercial enterprises to achieve health outcomes' (Doc. EB107/20) was submitted to the WHO Executive Board in January 2001. It replaced internal guidelines previously used by the Office of the Legal Counsel. The new Guidelines were reviewed during the Board session, although they were not intended as a formal WHO policy statement, but as internal guidance to the staff for dealing with problems of conflict of interest and other related problems.

The Guidelines recall that WHO's activities affect the commercial sector in broad ways through its public health guidance, its recommendations on regulatory standards, or other work that might influence product costs, market demand, or profitability of specific goods and services. Such activities include the setting of norms for quality, safety, and efficacy of pharmaceuticals and related promotional practices, dissemination of information on pharmaceuticals; provision of guidelines for diagnostics and treatment or advice that might affect the market for individual products and product categories; establishment of chemical safety standards, and formulation of nutritional guidelines. In developing relationships with commercial enterprises, WHO's reputation and values must be ensured. Scientific validity must not be compromised.

Assessment of companies would identify potential areas of conflict of interest. Relationships should be avoided with commercial enterprises whose activities are incompatible with WHO's work, such as the tobacco or arms industries. Relationships should contribute to improving public health; the public health gains should be commensurate with the time and expense involved in establishing and maintaining the relationship; relationships should be established on the basis of an exchange of letters or agreements indicating the contribution (financial or otherwise) that each of the parties brings to the relationship. Commercial enterprises will be expected to conform to WHO public health policies in the areas of food safety, chemical safety, ethical promotion of medicinal drug products, tobacco control, and others.

Specific guidance is given concerning cash donations, donations for clinical trials, for unspecified programme support, for WHO meetings, for financing staff salaries, for publications. Financing may not be accepted from commercial enterprises for activities leading to production of WHO guidelines or recommendations. No commercial advertisements may be placed in WHO publications. Contributions from commercial enterprises must be publicly acknowledged by WHO, normally through an insertion in the related documentation. Contributors may not use the results of WHO's work for commercial purposes or seek promotion from the fact that they have made a donation. Anonymous donations may not be accepted In determining the acceptability of large-scale donations of pharmaceuticals, there should be sound evidence of the safety and efficacy of such drug, and that the drug donation is not of a promotional nature, either with regard to the company itself, or by creating a demand for the drug which is not sustainable once the donation is ended. Secondments from commercial companies to WHO are acceptable for limited periods of time, but not from industries whose activities clearly conflict with WHO's mandate, such as arms and tobacco industries. The seconded person will follow the same rules of conduct as other WHO staff members. Collaborative research and development should, as a general rule, be undertaken only if WHO and the company concerned have concluded an agreement which ensures that the final product will ultimately be made widely available, including to the public sector of developing countries at a preferential price. In case of doubt as to the acceptability of an arrangement under the Guidelines, the Legal Counsel should be consulted, who may submit the case to the Committee on Private Sector Collaboration, an internal body first set up in the 1980s and re-established in 1998 (WHO, 2001b).

The review of the guidelines had caused both positive and negative comments. Most government representatives welcomed the issue of guidelines but expressed caution regarding the relations between WHO and the private sector. For the Indian representative, for instance, it had to be ensured that pharmaceutical companies and other commercial interests, notably the food industry, were not able to influence policy-making in WHO. As a certifying and standard-setting agency, WHO had a crucial role to play in lending legitimacy to any product or standard. In mobilizing resources, whether by accepting donations or by participating in product development, no compromise in the credibility and moral standing of WHO should be allowed (WHO, 2001a). In a letter of 10 January 2000 to WHO, the Director-General of IFPMA criticized the approach taken by WHO in the draft guidelines as overly defensive and suspicious of industry. They failed to address the key issues of concern to industry, namely confidentiality, respect for intellectual property and respect for market forces. At the January 2001 session of the Executive Board, however, the IFPMA representative said that IFPMA had no difficulties with the content and direction of the draft guidelines (WHO, 2001a).

At the same meeting, IBFAN's representative, speaking on behalf of Consumers International and HAI, felt that the guidelines fell short in critical areas. The cardinal principle of the guidelines should be complete accountability and transparency. However, they made no provision for an independent evaluation of potential donors and of their compliance with WHO standards and with international agreements on human rights, the environment, marketing and labour practices. The guidelines should include complete transparency on contractual agreements with all commercial enterprises and an assessment of potential donor companies. They should provide for the regular monitoring and evaluation of all private sector cooperation by an external body, including representatives of governments and civil society; a 'whistle-blowing' mechanism allowing staff to report problems without damage to their professional position or reputation and annual reports to the Executive Board on contractual agreements, their implementation and the public health outcomes achieved (WHO, 2001a).

The Director-General's response

Replying to some of the concerns expressed by governments and NGOs, the Director-General announced in December 2001 the following measures in complement to the approved guidelines (WHO, 2001d):

- proposals for any interaction between WHO and the private sector will need to be accompanied by a clear statement of purpose;
- guidelines to staff on handling interactions will be updated regularly to reflect experience and will include text on recognizing and avoiding conflict of interest. Although the guidelines are primarily for Secretariat use, they will continue to be available on the WHO headquarters web site for the information of Member States and the public;
- staff training modules on issues relating to private sector interaction and conflict of interest were being developed;
- declaration of interest forms were in use for all senior staff and WHO experts participating in meetings;
- a civil society initiative was in place to ensure input and engagement from NGOs;
- work was in progress on a tool to assess the good standing and practices of any company with whom interaction is envisaged;
- private sector interactions will be documented and reported to the Executive Board and Health Assembly, and will be available to the public.

Conclusion

The opening of WHO to the private sector, or rather, its recent expansion, brings both benefits and risks for the organization. The benefits are additional funding, allowing for more or expanded programmes, – the availability of other resources of private sector companies, including their research capacity, – the possibility of influencing the activities of these firms towards assistance and research of benefit to developing countries, – a better understanding of commercial enterprises' objectives and methods on the part of WHO staff, – a possible spillover of the result-oriented business partners' sense of initiative and creativity on the more bureaucratic WHO staff. The risks are an open or hidden domination of WHO's public health mission by the more powerful business firms, the possible neglect of priority areas and programmes, in particular for the developing countries, in favour of business-selected sectoral projects, – the cancellation, postponement or dilution of necessary standardization or regulation in the public health domain, – the possible 'commercialization' of WHO, bringing discredit to the mandatory independence, neutrality and scientific expertise of the organization, and curtailing its responsibility for the whole world, including the poorest countries and populations.

The expected benefits for commercial enterprises are clear: improving their profits through their publicized association with a respected global organization. The risks appear minimal: the loss of expected profits through donations and participation in voluntary programmes, or acceptance of some of WHO norms and standards, such as the priority given to generic drugs, to the detriment of brand medicines.

Assuming that WHO's interaction with the private sector is now acquired and growing, safeguards to the integrity of WHO's mission are needed. Essentially, these require setting up controls and insisting on transparency, the open acknowledgement of potential areas for conflict of interest. The organization should not initiate interaction with a commercial enterprise or business-related foundation without an independent assessment of its respect for WHO and UN standards. Once this interaction has been authorized, the business firm's behaviour should be monitored periodically, preferably by an independent body: violations should be publicly exposed and a decision taken as to whether the interaction should or not be continued. Research should be carried out on the effect of specific public/private partnerships on international public health, on the effectiveness of public health services in developing countries, on mortality and morbidity rates and other indicators, on the control or eradication of diseases, on the access to pharmaceuticals, to generic drugs, on the effect on equity.

The Director-General has taken a number of useful decisions in an attempt to control the potential risks of the expanded WHO interaction with the private sector. However, most of the measures announced in December 2001 are 'work in progress' and some are unclear: for instance, what 'civil society initiative' is in place, how does it function, does it satisfy NGOs claims? Is a tool (such as a Corporate Assessment instrument) to assess the good standing and practices of companies with whom interaction is envisaged now in place?

In spite of the Director-General's good intentions, it should be noted that all present controls are internal to the Organization, and therefore subject to potential conflicts of interest. Without doubting the Legal Counsel's competence and impartiality, nor those of the members of the WHO Committee on Private Sector Collaboration, they only represent one constituency, that of the secretariat: their assessments and conclusions will remain closed to public scrutiny, and thus lack transparency. Such difficult decisions as the rejection of a commercial company would best be taken on the basis of the assessment and recommendation by an independent external body including governments, the secretariat, NGOs and a federation of commercial enterprises, – or by a specially mandated interagency UN body, – or alternatively by a multinational audit firm specializing in 'social impact' evaluation and reporting. WHO would still retain its final decision. Such a body would also have an oversight responsibility on commercial enterprises' compliance with WHO and UN standards.

The following Chapters will give examples of WHO's consultation and cooperation with 'for-profit organizations' in specific areas and assess their results.

The first category involves the setting of policies by WHO, generally with the support of NGOs, which have been opposed by private sector firms or industries.

International Public Health

This has placed WHO in the uncomfortable position of being the target of NGOs for not being forceful enough, and the target of MNCs for threatening their interests (Part II).

The second category includes Public-Private Partnerships for Health, which have flourished especially during Dr Brundtland's mandate. Questions raised: why these partnerships? Is international public health a beneficiary or a loser in these alliances? (Part III).

The third category refers to WHO's rejection of cooperation with an industry, the tobacco industry, whose product is known to cause illness and death. In this case, WHO's policy is generally agreed by most Member States and strongly supported by NGOs. The public health enemy is named and the policy is not only non-cooperation, but a public fight against the industry (Part IV).

Notes

1 Dr Brundtland was three times Prime Minister of Norway. She chaired the World Commission on Environment and Development, whose report 'Our Common Future' was published in 1987. The Commission's recommendations led to the Rio Conference held in 1992.
2 For instance, in the period 1992–1993, 18.8% of the WHO budget, or $271 million, was spent on supplies and materials, furniture and equipment (Beigbeder, 1998, Table 9).
3 Letter from B. van der Heide, HAI, to Mr Denis Aitken, WHO, dated 22 December 1999.
4 Letter from E. Ram, World Vision to Mr Denis Aitken, WHO, dated 23 December 1999.
5 *In re* MOORE, Judgment 1405, 1 February 1995.
6 *The Lancet,* Vol. 354, No. 9181, p. 787, – *La Revue Prescrire,* Tome 19, No. 195, May 1999, and letter from Chief Editor, *Prescrire,* dated 16 April 1999.
7 Letter from Chairman, ICDB to WHO Director General dated 12 January 2000.
8 Letter from Mr B. van der Heide, Coordinator HAI Europe to Dr Brundtland dated 18 May 1999. Dr Brundtland's letter of June 1999 is on www.haiweb.org/news/sponsorship.response.html, 16 February 2001, – Consumers International's response of May 1999 is in WHO Doc. EB105/SR/2, 24 January 2000, p. 16.
9 HAI's letter of 19 June 1996 to the President of the World Bank, Bank's reply of 27 June 1996, – R. Laing's letter of 2 July 1996 (Boston University School of Public Health) to the President of the World Bank.

PART II
SETTING INTERNATIONAL PUBLIC HEALTH POLICY

Chapter 3

The Promotion of Breastfeeding

In 1981, the World Health Assembly adopted the International Code of Marketing of Breast-milk Substitutes in the form of a recommendation under Article 23 of the WHO Constitution. For the first time, a WHO initiative collided with major business interests, raising violent polemics between NGOs and infant food industry multinational companies.[1]

The adoption of the Code

Paediatrician Dr Cecily Williams, later the first Director of WHO's Maternal and Child Health Programme, first raised the alarm on infant feeding in her 1939 address to the Singapore Rotary Club entitled 'Milk and Murder':

> If you are a legal purist, you may wish me to change the title of this address to Milk and Manslaughter. But if your lives were as embittered as mine is, by seeing day after day this massacre of the innocents by unsuitable feeding, then I believe you would feel as I do that misguided progaganda on infant feeding should be punished as the most criminal form of sedition, and that these deaths should be regarded as murder (Allain, 1986).

International action to deal with this problem started thirty years later, in December 1969. A working group of the Protein Advisory Group (PAG) of the UN System (formerly the FAO/UNICEF/WHO Group) was then set up in Bogota to review the conditions of infant nutrition, *in utero* and during the first months of life, in various regions of the Third World. Specialists from universities, governments or industry who met on this occasion had the same concern: there was a decline in breastfeeding, without a clear indication of its causes. However, there was a feeling that the over-aggressive promotion of breast-milk substitutes played an important role in this phenomenon. At this stage, the participants to the PAG meeting tried to find a ground for agreement in order to avoid debatable commercial practices. All participants agreed on two points:

- The superiority of breast-feeding;
- The high quality of substitute products offered by industry.

However, the industry representatives rejected any relationship between the availability and promotion of infant formula and the decline in breastfeeding.

The PAG working group met again in Paris in 1972 and published its conclusions in a document called *Declaration 23* which defined precisely the responsibilities of governments and industry in fighting against the progressive decline of breastfeeding. A spirit of cooperation then prevailed and a proposal was made to initiate a lasting effort in this direction. The debate hardened in 1973, when the *New Internationalist* published an article implicating directly breast-milk substitutes sold by large companies, including Nestlé: the cover of the periodical showed a child's grave on which was placed an empty feeding bottle and the packing of 'Lactogen', a Nestlé product. The *New Internationalist*, sponsored by three humanitarian NGOs, Oxfam, Christian Aid and Third World First, accused the manufacturers of selling off in the Third World poor quality products, of neglecting the formulation of clear instructions to illiterate mothers, of disguising their sales persons as nurses in order to sell their preparations at any price to young mothers.

The dialogue was totally broken in 1974 when Mike Muller, a British journalist working for the humanitarian organization War on Want, published during a press conference in London the report on the discussions he had had with Nestlé officials. The title of this report – Nestlé, The Baby Killer – summarized in a provocative way the basic idea of its author: the promotion of breast-milk substitutes had a direct incidence on infant malnutrition in the Third World. It was therefore necessary to 'de-commercialize' all breast-milk substitutes, and even suppress the educational instructions necessary for the proper utilization of the products. The Swiss 'Dritte Welt Arbeitsgruppe' (the Third World's Working Group) adapted the War on Want publication and changed its title to *Nestlé kills Babies*. Nestlé sued for libel and the group was later ordered to pay compensation for defamation, as the Court in Bern had found no direct causal relation between the sale or distribution of powdered milk and the death of babies fed with the company's product.

The verbal and media escalation went on during the following years. Some of the significant stages of the developing crisis follow:

- 1975, the manufacturers create a new association, the International Council of Infant Food Industries (ICIFI), whose mandate was to regulate more efficiently their commercial activities in the Third World and to act as the spokesperson of the industry in the conflict;
- in the same year, the NGO activists created *Infact* (Infant Formula Action Coalition) joining individuals and organizations committed to the anti-producers' campaign;
- also in 1975, the campaign started in the USA, with the support of a few religious organizations which managed to mobilize part of the middle class;
- in 1977, beginning of the boycott launched in the USA by *Infact* against Nestlé products;
- in 1978: holding of a televised Congressional Committee Hearing chaired by Senator Robert Kennedy, which exposed in front of millions of televiewers the conflict activists-industry. During this parliamentary investigation the proposal was made to entrust WHO with the organization of a conference during which an ethical marketing code would be elaborated.

In October 1979, WHO and UNICEF convened a Meeting on Infant and Young Child Feeding which was attended by 150 representatives of WHO Member States, organizations of the UN system, professional associations, scientists, the infant food industry and NGOs. Among the latter, *Infact*, War on Want and Dritte Welt

Arbeitsgruppe had been among the most committed activists. From the beginning, the industry representatives opposed the contents of the working document issued by WHO and UNICEF to serve as a basis for the discussions. In their view, this document reflected the activists' main claims, which led the industry representatives to draft their own document. The very stormy meeting reached a number of conclusions showing the incompatibility of the viewpoints of the participants. The tenuous, perhaps impossible, dialogue between manufacturers and activists was again broken. Following the meeting, the activists established the International Baby Food Action Network (IBFAN), joining those groups including *Infact* which intended to continue the boycott campaign. On its side, ICIFI issued a voluntary code for manufacturers, as a preferred alternative to an international code, which was also meant to facilitate the formulation of national regulations by governments, or to only serve as a guide for industry firms.

One of the recommendations of the 1979 meeting was to request WHO and UNICEF to prepare, in consultation with all the parties concerned, an international code of marketing of breast-milk substitutes. In 1980, the World Health Assembly endorsed that recommendation and requested the WHO Director-General to prepare an international code, either in the form of a regulation or as a recommendation (Res. WHA33.32). From May to December, four drafts were discussed: the final text was the result of numerous compromises.

Beside the discussions on the contents of the Code, its legal form was another contested issue. The Assembly had ruled out the use of a treaty, convention or agreement under Article 19 of the WHO Constitution. Alternatives were either a regulation or a recommendation. A regulation may be considered as 'quasi-legislative' as, after its adoption by the Assembly, it comes into force for all Member States after due notice has been given of its adoption by the Assembly 'except for such Members as may notify the Director-General of rejection or reservations within the period stated in the notice' (Art. 22). A recommendation adopted under Article 23 of the WHO Constitution does not have binding effect. However, recommendations 'carry moral or political weight, as they constitute the judgement on a health issue of the collective membership of the highest international body in the field of health' (Shubber, 1985: 881, 884).

Hoping for a unanimous support from Member States, in a failed attempt to override the US opposition to international regulation of trade, the WHO Executive Board recommended the adoption of a non-binding recommendation. Its representative pleaded for consensus:

> We are not today dealing with an economic issue of particular importance only to one or a few Member States. We are dealing with a health issue of essential importance to all Member States, and particularly to developing nations, and of importance to the children of the world and thus to all future generations (Richter, 2001: 67).

The World Health Assembly adopted the Code as a recommendation on 21 May 1981, as a 'minimum requirement' to be applied 'in its entirety'. One hundred and eighteen Member States voted in favour of the Code, the USA voted against and three countries (Argentina, Japan and the Republic of Korea) abstained.

Contents of the Code

The Code was developed to promote the exclusive feeding of breast-milk from birth to four or six months of age and to protect mothers and health workers from commercial pressures by manufacturers of breast-milk substitutes. The Code affirms that breast-feeding provides the ideal food for the healthy growth and development of infants; it forms a unique biological and emotional basis for the health of both mother and child; moreover, breast-milk has anti-infective properties, which help to protect infants against disease (WHO, 1981:10). On the other hand, the premature and improper use of breast-milk substitutes may lead to sickness and mortality in infants.

The formal aim of the Code is '... to contribute to the provision of safe and adequate nutrition for infants, by the protection and promotion of breast-feeding, and by ensuring the proper use of breast-milk substitutes, when these are necessary, on the basis of adequate information and through appropriate marketing and distribution' (Art. 1).

The Code expressly recognizes the need for breast-milk substitutes when the mother is unable to breast-feed her infant, for one reason or another, and emphasizes the constructive role played by the manufacturers and distributors of these products (Preamble of the Code).

To achieve its aim, the Code prescribes the following principles:

- Prohibition of advertising and promotion to the general public of products within the scope of the Code, through television, radio, newspapers, magazines, posters, or in any other form; it includes brand and non-brand, direct and indirect advertising and promotion; also prohibited are point-of-sale advertising, or any other promotion device to induce sales directly to the consumer at the retail revel, such as special displays, discount coupons, special sales, loss-leaders and tie-in sales for products within the scope of the Code (Art. 5.1 and 5.3).
- Prohibition of the giving of samples: manufacturers and distributors should not provide, directly or indirectly, samples of products to pregnant women, mothers or members of their families, if the purpose of giving of samples is promotional (Art. 5.2, 5.3).
- Prohibition of gifts and other inducements, such as the direct gift of breast-milk substitutes to the mother, the health worker, or some national institutions (Art. 5.4).
- Restriction on the use of bonuses and quotas as sales incentives for marketing personnel of manufacturers and distributors (Art. 8.1).
- Article 4.1 places responsibility for education and information on the governments.
- Consumer protection: requirements as to the quality and labelling of products (Art. 9.2, 9.3, 9.4, 10).
- Governments are responsible for the implementation of the Code through adoption of national legislation, regulations or other suitable measures (Art. 11.1). They may seek the cooperation of WHO, UNICEF or other UN agencies in meeting this requirement.

- Monitoring the application of the Code lies with governments acting individually and collectively through WHO. Private individuals, NGOs, and professional groups and institutions are responsible for drawing the attention of manufacturers and distributors to activities which are incompatible with the principles and aim of the Code, so that appropriate action may be taken. Finally, the Code adds to these external monitoring processes a self-monitoring responsibility on the part of the manufacturers and distributors to monitor their marketing practices according to the principles and aim of the Code, and for taking steps to ensure that their conduct at every level conforms to them (Art. 11.2, 11.3, 11.4).

After the Code

Following the adoption of the Code in 1981, a few policy statements confirmed and reinforced its aim and principles of promotion of breastfeeding and prevention of inappropriate marketing of breast-milk substitutes.

In 1989, WHO and UNICEF published a *Joint Statement Protecting, Promoting and Supporting Breastfeeding: The Special Role of Maternity Services*. The Statement lists 'Ten Steps to Successful Breastfeeding', as shown in Presentation 3.1. These were based on research evidence and on mothers' experience of what made breastfeeding go well.

The Convention on the Rights of the Child was adopted by the UN General Assembly on 20 November 1989. It entered into force in 1990. A legally binding human rights instrument, it was ratified by 191 out of 193 governments: the USA was a signatory but is not a State Party. Somalia, a failed State, was the other exception. The Convention recognizes, *inter alia*, the need for access to and availability of both support and information concerning the use of basic knowledge of child health and nutrition, and the advantages of breastfeeding for all segments of society, in particular parents and children (Art.24).

At its 88th session in June 2000, the International Labour Conference adopted the Maternity Protection Convention, 2000 (No. 183) and Maternity Protection Recommendation, 2000 (No. 191). With the participation of WHO, the Convention was strengthened, in part, through an increase in the entitlement to a minimum length of maternity leave from 12 to 14 weeks and reinforcement of the entitlement to paid breastfeeding breaks (WHO, 2001e).

In July 1990, a new meeting on the promotion of breastfeeding was convened by WHO and UNICEF at the International Child Development Centre in Florence, Italy. The meeting issued the 'Innocenti Declaration', which called for the creation of an environment 'enabling all women to practice exclusive breastfeeding , and all infants to feed exclusively on breast-milk from birth to four to six months of age'. In September 1990, the World Summit for Children issued a Declaration including a provision supporting breastfeeding. In 1991, a new international NGO consortium was formed: the World Alliance for Breastfeeding Action.

The 'Ten Steps' were then expanded into the Global Criteria for the Baby-Friendly Hospital Initiative, launched by WHO and UNICEF in June 1991. Hospitals joining this programme promise not to accept 'free' or low-cost supplies of breast-milk substitutes from infant food manufacturers and distributors and pledge to redesign their services so as to create an environment in which mothers who choose to do so can breastfeed (Black, 1996:77, 78).

Presentation 3.1

Ten Steps to Successful Breastfeeding

Every facility providing maternity services and care for newborn infants should have a written breastfeeding policy that is routinely communicated to all health care staff.

1. Train all health care staff in skills necessary to implement this policy.
2. Inform all pregnant women about the benefits and management of breastfeeding.
3. Help mothers initiate breastfeeding within half an hour of birth.
4. Show mothers how to breastfeed, and how to maintain lactation even if they should be separated from their infants.
5. Give newborn infants no food or drink other than breastmilk, unless medically indicated.
6. Practice rooming-in – that is, allow mothers and infants to remain together – 24 hours a day.
7. Encourage breastfeeding on demand.
8. Give no artificial teats or pacifiers (also called dummies or soothers) to breastfeeding infants.
9. Foster the establishment of breastfeeding support groups and refer mothers to them on discharge from the hospital or clinic.

Source: Joint WHO/UNICEF document published in 1989 by WHO, Geneva.

By 2002, Baby-Friendly programmes had been launched in 171 countries: 16,000 hospitals were implementing the Initiative's criteria in 125 countries, and more were designated each year. However, standards were not always maintained, the global number of facilities designated 'baby friendly' appeared to have reached a plateau. Some countries reported weakened commitment, particularly in private and university teaching hospitals, having interpreted diminishing resources from WHO and UNICEF as a sign of reduced international interest (Armstrong, 1999, WHO, 2002c).

Monitoring the implementation of the Code

In accordance with Art. 11.6 of the Code, governments should send an annual report to the WHO Director-General on the action they have taken to implement the Code. The Director-General then reports in even years to the World Health Assembly on the status of implementation of the Code by governments (Art. 11.7). An Assembly resolution generally endorses the Director-General's report, confirms the validity of the Code's guidance and acknowledges the efforts made by WHO, UNICEF and other international partners in supporting its implementation. This biannual exercise is an occasion given to both NGOs and industry representatives at the Executive Board and the Assembly to give their own appraisal of the value of the Code and of its implementation by both governments and the industry. However, these reports do not include specific information, country by country, of the degree of compliance with the Code. For instance, the only information given to the Assembly in May 2002 was that, since the adoption of the Code, 162 of WHO's 191 Member States had reported on their action to give effect to the Code's principles and aims (WHO, 2002c). WHO does not provide information as to the degree of compliance with the Code of its industry partners.

Monitoring reports have been issued mainly by experts and professional groups and by IBFAN. All reports point to widespread violations of the Code's prescriptions by the manufacturers and distributors.

In a report published by the British Medical Journal (BMJ) in 1998 (Taylor, 1998), an epidemiological study carried out in four countries showed that one tenth of all mothers interviewed and a quarter of all facilities visited had received free samples of milk, bottles, or teats – none of them for research purposes. Violating information was received by 30 percent of health facilities, and 11 percent of health workers surveyed had received gifts, three quarters of which bore a company's brand name. The study was designed to measure the prevalence of violations of the Code using randomly sampled groups of women, health workers, and health facilities in the four cities of the four countries. No funding, support, or advice was received from the manufacturers of breast-milk substitutes or organizations forming part of the IBFAN network. It was therefore a scientific study carried out independently of organizations directly concerned with the issue.

In its 1998 Report on 'Breaking the Rules, Stretching the Rules', IBFAN revealed violations of the Code during a 31-country survey carried out between January and September 1997 (IBFAN, 1998). The survey results showed that in nearly every participating country, the main producers of infant formula and other breast-milk substitutes did not comply with the requirements set by the World Health Assembly. The most significant finding was the industry's continued focus on the health care system, i.e. hospital maternity units. Mothers, health workers and hospitals still received free samples and supplies from numerous companies, headed by Abbott Ross, Mead Johnson, Nestlé and Wyeth. Companies were still using posters, clocks, calendars and gifts to mothers and health workers as a way to promote products.

Similar results were reported in IBFAN's 2001 'Breaking the Rules' report. The monitoring results covered 16 transnational baby food companies and 13 manufacturers of bottles and teats. Health care facilities continued to be the most widely used and most efficient avenue for companies to reach mothers. Mothers in maternity units receive promotional material such as booklets and leaflets on infant feeding, free samples and gifts such as car stickers, baby records, coupons, bottle tags and towels. Company names or brand names appear on posters, clocks and calendars. Almost all companies included in the survey provided free infant formula to health care facilities, and free samples to health workers. None of those companies was complying fully with the labelling requirements of the Code.

Article 11.3 of the Code makes manufacturers and distributors responsible for monitoring their marketing practices according to the principles and aim of the Code and for taking steps to ensure that their conduct at every level conforms to them. Nestlé submitted to the WHO Director-General in July 1999 a report entitled 'Nestlé implementation of the WHO Code (International Code of Marketing of Breast-milk Substitutes) Official Response of Governments'. In a legal evaluation of this report, a Consultant to IBFAN and to the Geneva Infant Feeding Association (GIFA) submitted that neither the criteria used by Nestlé for its self-monitoring, nor its approach to self-monitoring was in conformity with the Code (IBFAN, 2000). The criterion used by Nestlé was what the governments endorse and accept as their interpretation of the Code in their countries. Moreover, instead of investigating and inspecting the marketing practices of its own agents, Nestlé approached health ministries in 54 Member States of WHO and asked them to inform it of any violation of the Code. They were also asked to confirm, in writing, Nestlé's compliance with the Code. Nestlé then used these replies as written evidence of its compliance with the Code. UNICEF Executive Director Carol Bellamy expressed similar reservations to the claim that the Nestlé report fulfilled the company's obligation under Article 11.3 of the Code. In a letter of 31 December 1999, she stated that the Code requires that both governments and manufacturers establish distinct and separate monitoring systems: 'Obtaining certificates of Code compliance where monitoring is not taking place would not seem to us an appropriate basis for such a claim' (Bellamy, 1999a).

The misconduct of commercial enterprises

The WHO 'Global Strategy on infant and young child feeding', endorsed by resolution WHA55.25 by the World Health Assembly on 18 May 2002 (WHO, 2002) states, in its paragraph 44, that all manufacturers and distributors of products within the scope of the Code 'should ensure that their conduct at every level conforms to the Code, subsequent relevant Health Assembly resolutions, and national measures that have been adopted to give effect to both'.

Far from maintaining such a conduct, reports from researchers and NGOs show a pattern of opposition, on the part of commercial enterprises, to the full implementation of the Code. The reasons are obvious: commercial enterprises are profit-driven, and the Code is liable to limit or decrease their profits. As stated bluntly by Helmut Maucher, former Chief Executive Officer of Nestlé, 'Ethical decisions that injure a firm's ability to compete are actually immoral'.[2]

Attacked by NGO groups, the baby-food industry fought back by affirming that international regulation was an unwanted interference in the free market. Before the adoption of the Code, in a testimony at a US Senate hearing, Nestlé and three US companies declared that they did not intend to abide by the recommendations of the 1979 WHO/UNICEF meeting. Writing as President of ICIFI in 1981, Nestlé Vice President Ernest Saunders described the draft marketing Code as unacceptable, restrictive, irrelevant and unworkable (IBFAN, 2001b).

After the adoption of the Code, a few commercial enterprises have adopted voluntary codes, as weaker substitutes to the WHO/UNICEF Code. They have used trade threats to developing countries in order to weaken national legislation implementing the Code. Richter (2001: 127–129) recalls that Guatemala had to weaken its law in 1995 after extensive legal and trade pressure from the US company Gerber (now a subsidiary of the Swiss Novartis). The industry also opposed the introduction of national legislation in Costa Rica on the grounds that a proposed bill would establish non-tariff barriers to trade in violation of GATT agreements and would interfere with industry's constitutional freedom of speech. Similar threats were addressed to the Zimbabwean Parliament, which still passed its legislation in May 1998. One particularly odious tactic has been to threaten critics in order to silence them. Richter (2001: 152, 157, 158, 174) refers to critics losing their jobs, threats of physical harm, including death threats. Critics are labelled as communists, anti-free marketeers, corporation haters, in order to discredit them.

Other issues

The duration of exclusive breastfeeding

The first World Health Assembly resolution on this subject, adopted in May 1978, only recognized that 'during the first few months of life' breastfeeding was the safest and most appropriate way to feed infants and that it should be maintained as long as possible (Res. WHA31.47). Since 1979, the WHO recommendation for the duration of exclusive breastfeeding has been 'four to six months'. The Innocenti Declaration of 1990 recommended that infants should be fed exclusively on breast-milk from birth to four to six months.

Since 1993, key UNICEF publications have recommended exclusive breastfeeding as follows: 'Breast-milk alone is the best possible food and drink for a baby. No other food or drink is needed for about the first six months of life. A variety of additional foods is necessary when a child is about six months old, but breastfeeding should continue well into the second year of a child's life and for longer if possible' (UNICEF, 1993). The same formulation – for about the first six months of life – was used in a UNICEF publication issued in 1999 (UNICEF, 1999b).

WHO was slower than UNICEF in changing the duration of exclusive breastfeeding from 'four to six months' to about six months. In 1994, the World Health Assembly recommended the introduction of appropriate complementary feeding practices 'from the age of about six months', thus indirectly recognizing that exclusive breastfeeding should be fostered for about the first six months (Res. 47.5).

In March 2000, WHO organized a consultation of 28 experts to assess infant and young child feeding policies, review key interventions, and formulate a comprehensive strategy for the next decade. During the meeting, the experts suggested the urgent need to state 'about six months of age' as the best recommendation for the age of introduction of complementary foods to babies. Inconsistencies in WHO publications between 'four to six months' and 'about six months' were confusing and needed resolution. However, the WHO technical staff refused to allow such discussion during the meeting. WHO's position was that research was being undergone and would be examined in 2001. 'Because this research is under way, both the consultation's terms of reference and the selection of participants precluded in depth discussion of the optimal duration of exclusive breastfeeding' (Ferriman, 2000). During the 53rd Assembly, in May 2000, the Brazilian delegation proposed a resolution in favour of exclusive breastfeeding for six months. The resolution did not pass.

Taking into account the findings of the WHO expert consultation held in Geneva in March 2001, the World Health Assembly finally adopted in May the 'exclusive breastfeeding for six months' formulation as a 'global public health recommendation' (Res. WHA54.2). A year later, the Assembly endorsed a Global strategy on infant and young child feeding which also supported, in part, 'exclusive breastfeeding for six months and continuous breastfeeding up to two years of age or beyond' (Res. WHA55.25).

IBFAN blamed the WHO Secretariat for trying to postpone the earlier resolution of this issue. IBFAN had maintained that the 'delay resulted mainly in large profits gained by infant food manufacturers from sales of complementary foods for two additional months of complementary feeding' (IBFAN, 2002). There is however no evidence that the WHO Secretariat purposefully delayed the resolution of the issue because of pressures from the baby food industry. The WHO delay can be explained by the need to have a clear finding from the expert group and possibly, bureaucratic hurdles.

The six-month recommendation applies to populations as a public health policy recommendation. Adaptation to the needs of the individual should still be done one by one, through individual case management.

Breastfeeding by HIV-positive mothers

The promotion of breastfeeding has met a recent, lethal obstacle. Each year, more than 600,000 infants become infected by HIV/AIDS, mainly in developing countries. Since the beginning of the HIV epidemic, an estimated 5.1 million children worldwide have been infected with HIV. Mother-to-child transmission is responsible for more than 90 percent of these infections. Two-thirds are believed to occur during pregnancy and delivery, and about one- third through breastfeeding.

According to a Technical Consultation held in Geneva from 11–13 October 2000, up to 20 percent of infants born to HIV-positive mothers may acquire HIV through breastfeeding (UNAIDS, 2000). The meeting concluded that the guidelines issued in 1998 by WHO, UNICEF and UNAIDS remained valid. An HIV-infected woman should receive counselling, which includes information about the risks and benefits of different infant feeding options, and specific guidance in selecting the option most likely to be suitable for her situation. The final decision should be the woman's, and she should be supported in her choice. For HIV-positive women who choose to breastfeed, exclusive breastfeeding is recommended for the first months of life, and should be discontinued when an alternative form of feeding becomes feasible.

In May 2001, the World Health Assembly recognized the need for independent research on the balance of risk of HIV transmission through breastfeeding compared with the risk of not breastfeeding (Res. WHA54.2). It also recognized that when replacement feeding is acceptable, feasible, affordable, sustainable and safe, avoidance of all breastfeeding by HIV-positive women is recommended. Otherwise, exclusive breastfeeding is recommended during the first months of life: those who choose other options should be encouraged to use them free from commercial influences.

Conclusion

In 2002, 21 years after the adoption of the Code, WHO has reported that malnutrition has been responsible, directly or indirectly, for 60 percent of the 10.9 million deaths annually among children under five (WHO, 2002d: 4). Well over two-thirds of these deaths, often associated with inappropriate feeding practices, occur during the first year of life. No more than 35 percent of infants worldwide are exclusively breastfed during the first four months of life: complementary feeding begins too early or too late, and foods are often nutritionally inadequate and unsafe. Hence the need for renewed efforts at both national and international levels to apply the Code's prescriptions.

Progress is dependent on the support of a cluster of actors: governments, health workers, families and communities, international organizations, NGOs and associations, and the baby food industry.

Governments are primarily responsible for defining and applying a national policy and regulation on infant and young child feeding in accordance with the prescriptions of the Code. Governments are however divided over this issue. The USA has voted against the Code and is, at times, applying political and economic pressures on developing countries in the process of adopting their own policies and legislation in line with the Code. European Union policies on infant feeding fail to meet the minimum requirements of the Code and World Health Assembly resolutions. In October 2001, IBFAN asked for confirmation from the European Commission on Trade to the following statement: 'For the optimum health in infants in both Europe and Third World Countries EU legislation should be brought in line with the International Code and subsequent relevant Resolutions'. The Commission's answer was non-committal: 'To the extent that the EU and its Member States subscribe to them – to a large extent, these are issues of Member State competence' (IBFAN, 2001c). The UK government was one of the main supporters for the adoption of the Code and for later World Health Assembly resolutions. The UK law, adopted in 1995, contains important safeguards such as a ban on free samples and free supplies. However, advertising of baby foods to the public is allowed, although prohibited by the Code. As a more positive sign, in January 1999, the European Parliament adopted a resolution calling for controls on European businesses operating in developing countries. These hearings may lead to a Directive making companies answerable in the law courts of Europe if they break international standards on health, the environment and human rights (IBFAN 1999).

EU Member States adopt the Code, endorse the WHO Global Strategy and World Health Assembly resolutions, and then shy away from implementing all the principles and practices set by UN bodies at the regional or national level. Is this due to a lack of understanding of and interest for the Code, a lack of political will, and/or pressures from the industry?

The governments of developing nations are more exposed to direct pressures from the multinational companies, with the support of their home countries. Some of them have been the object of trade threats to limit or abandon their legislation.

WHO and the more outspoken UNICEF have facilitated the birth of the Code and are its guardians. Even though the Code is only a recommendation, and not a binding legal instrument, it has set desirable standards, which carry scientific, technical and moral weight. Later World Health Assembly resolutions, based on scientific findings, have further added to the Code's authority. However, WHO, as an intergovernmental organization, is loath to blame individual governments for a lack of compliance with the Code. It maintains an uneasy relationship with NGOs, as keen supporters of WHO standards and necessary helpers at the local level, but also as uncomfortably strident voices denouncing the 'devious ways' of the multinational companies.

The baby food industry is not an adversary for WHO, as the tobacco industry is. However, it cannot be a *bona fide* partner in view of its different objectives, its profit-making nature. The industry's strength and financial power require that WHO keeps its distance from its influence and exercises caution in joint consultation groups, particularly in scientific assessments and norm-setting.[3]

Baby food corporations pretend to accept the Code's prescriptions but fail to comply with them in their entirety. When caught red handed, they tend to deny ill-doing. They have developed weak codes as an inadequate substitute for the Code. They do not monitor their own practices in relation to the Code's requirements.

Their basic objective, maximizing sales and profits, their promotion of unrestricted free trade and of a self-asserted 'freedom of commercial speech' are in direct conflict with the Code's aim to protect breastfeeding and limit the exercise of marketing.

NGOs have played an essential role in the adoption of the Code, in supporting WHO and UNICEF and in monitoring the implementation of the Code. They publicize the result of their surveys and research and effectively use the same 'shame' tactics vs. multinationals for their violations of the Code's prescriptions as done by Amnesty International for human rights violations.

Monitoring only by NGOs is however not sufficient. WHO should take a more assertive role. The organization could set up an independent group of international experts who would review and assess periodically the compliance with the Code of national governments and of baby food companies. As for a WHO Expert Committee, the group's report would then be submitted by the WHO Secretariat to the Executive Board and World Health Assembly.

The main obstacle to the implementation of the Code is caused by the ambiguous stance of the baby food industry. One could hope that, seeing the damage done to its public image, CEOs of two or three major producers would solemnly and publicly declare that their firms will, from now on, fully abide by the Code's prescriptions, and by further recommendations of the World Health Assembly, in their entirety. They would then publicly give precise instructions to their subsidiaries and agents, and apply sanctions to those subsidiaries and agents charged with non-compliance. Their own self-monitoring would then be provided periodically to the UN organizations concerned, NGOs and the general public.

This hope is however unlikely to be satisfied. In the circumstances, pressures on the industry by WHO, UNICEF, health professionals, NGOs and the media remain as necessary as ever.

Notes

1   The principal reference on this topic is Judith Richter's '*Holding Corporations Accountable*' (2001), a comprehensive study and assessment of corporate involvement in the infant feeding issue, which includes an extensive bibliography. Of particular interest is Dr S. Shubber's book on '*The International Code of Marketing of Breast-milk Substitutes: An International Measure to Protect and Promote Breast-feeding* (1998): Dr Shubber is a former Senior Legal Officer in WHO.
2   Cited in the *New Internationalist*, March 2001 and quoted in the Executive Summary of IBFAN's 'Breaking the Rules 2001'.
3   For instance, Nestlé SA, the largest food company in the world, posted a profit of 5.66 billion Swiss Francs ($3.76 billion) in first half of 2002 (*IHT*, 22 August 2002). Its annual promotion budget for all its products was $7.9 billion in 2001 (IBFAN, 2001). In comparison, WHO's total budget for 2001 was less than $1 billion, UNICEF's total expenditures for the same year was approximately $1.2 billion.

Chapter 4

Essential Drugs and the Pharmaceutical Industry

On 19 April 2001, the Pharmaceutical Manufacturers Association of South Africa and 39 multinational pharmaceutical companies unconditionally dropped their case against the South African government. The South African government had passed the Medicines and Related Substances Control Amendment Act ('Medicines Act') in 1997, which allowed importation of affordable medicines and increased use of generic drugs. This legislation was opposed by the US government and the European Union, in support of their pharmaceutical companies, objecting to the legitimization of parallel importing and compulsory licensing, claiming that it was at variance with World Trade Organization obligations (Thomas, 2002). The US government applied trade pressures against the South African government, while the 39 pharmaceutical companies submitted their case to the Pretoria High Court in 1998. The industry's court action was widely and publicly denounced by 140 NGOs from 130 countries who had signed the global 'Drop the Case' petition (MSF, 2001).

This unexpected success of a developing country, with the support of NGOs, for the protection of their patients' rights, marked the 'intrusion' of public health concerns in trade negotiations, triggering the necessary interference of WHO in international trade. The main issue is, in simple terms: should there be a 'health exception' in the rules of international and national trade?

The NGOs' essential pressures

The South African victory would not have been obtained without the effective pressures of local, national and international NGOs, relayed by the media. International NGOs have engaged in a long-term effort to broaden the access of poor populations to essential medicines, to obtain significant price reductions on brand medicine from pharmaceutical companies, to promote the production and sale of generic drugs. The major international NGOs lobby governments, the governing bodies and secretariats of intergovernmental organizations such as WHO, UNICEF, the World Bank, WTO. They issue press releases, research papers. MSF founded its 'Access to Essential Medicines Campaign' using the funds received when the organization won the 1999 Nobel Peace Prize. Oxfam's 'Cut the Cost Campaign' was launched in February 2001. One early objective of the campaign was to help activists in South Africa to force the 39 pharmaceutical companies to drop their lawsuit against the government. Oxfam's campaign then backed Brazilian NGOs in making the US withdraw their complaint at the WTO over Brazil's patent laws. MSF and Oxfam have joined with Third World Network, Consumer Project on Technology, Consumers International, Health Action International and The

Network in supporting the developing countries' claims at and following the WTO Doha meeting in November 2001. CorpWatch and Human Rights Watch are also on their side.

The industry's stance

Industry's leaders submit that private business has a right to be profit-oriented, to protect its investments, and to be compensated for innovation. Without industry funding, important advances in disease prevention and treatment would not have occurred. In the words of Lee Goldman, chairman of the Department of Medicine, University of California at San Francisco, 'companies translate biological advances into usable products for patients. They do it for a profit motive, but they do it, and it needs to be done' (Bodenheimer, 2000). Patents should be respected. Their purpose is to encourage innovation, and thus growth, by creating an incentive for inventors to disclose the details of their inventions in exchange for a time-limited monopoly on exploitation. Raymond Gilmartin, CEO, Merck & Co.Ltd. dismissed the impact of patents and their prices as the prime cause of lack of health protection in developing countries. He said recently: 'We know that patents are not significant barriers to access [of patients to medicines], because in many countries in need, patents do not exist'. He added: 'many essential drugs that are required for treatment are available off patents. We have also demonstrated that price alone is not the answer to access. By providing HIV/AIDS medicines at prices from which we make no profit in the world's poorest countries, we have been able to reach more people – but not the millions that are in need' (Gilmartin, 2002). Replying to attacks against the industry, an IFPMA representative said that, first the pharmaceutical industry creates and develops the medicines that save and improve the lives of millions of people. Furthermore, the companies are engaged in more than 50 partnerships in collaboration with WHO and others. Among these, the Accelerating Access Initiative on the HIV/AIDS crisis, – the Medicines for Malaria Venture, the Global Alliance for Vaccine and Immunization. One company is offering a drug for opportunistic HIV/AIDS infections at no cost in the 50 least developed countries. Since 1998, the industry has contributed $1.9 billion in donations of products to developing countries through partnerships (Bale, 2002).

The industry's image problem

A Novartis representative recognized in October 2002 that 'Big Pharma' suffers from an image problem (Leisinger, 2002). For him, one of the reasons for which the industry is the focus of public uneasiness is this sector's comparatively high profits in a world shaped by increasing income inequalities: 'in a world where the differences in infant, child, and maternal mortality probably represent the most obscene aspect of the North-South conflict, societies expect industry to do their share in creating better access to "medical care", including medicines'. However, the industry underlines that those most responsible for providing remedies to this inequality are the governments of poor countries and the institutions in industrial countries responsible for development cooperation. The former need substantial improvements in the area of good governance (stopping corruption and waste of scarce resources). The latter have forgotten about the 'peace dividend' which was to follow the end of the Cold War. Additional domestic and international financing to buy the drugs and to build effective health and supply systems are required.

The image problem cannot be dismissed so easily. The law suit in South Africa did not project a compassionate image of the industry: the case was abandoned only as a result of public pressures from NGOs and the fear of a lasting negative effect on the companies. While useful research is carried out by the companies, purchasing power and expected profits, not health needs, define drug research priorities. MSF (2002a) reports that only 10 per cent of global health research money is devoted to conditions that account for 90 per cent of the global disease burden. In 2001, the total global expenditure on health research was estimated at $60–70 billion. Of this, less than $70 million was spent on developing new and badly needed treatments for malaria, tuberculosis, African sleeping sickness and kala-azar. Other allegations cast a negative cloud on the industry, or on specific companies: efforts by drug companies 'to suppress, spin, and obfuscate findings that do not suit their commercial purposes' (The Lancet, 2001), gifts to doctors to market their products, inappropriate drug donations, threats to individuals who are perceived to challenge their interests.[1] Western-based companies increasingly export medical experiments to developing countries, where patients are plentiful and government oversight is weak or non-existent. According to the International Herald Tribune (Pear/Oppel, 2002), executives from Wyeth, Bristol-Myers Squibb Co., Eli Lilly Co. and Merck & Co. met near Washington, D.C. in November 2002 to discuss specific ways to leverage their more than $30 million investment in helping elect allies in the US Congress. Pervasive themes were how to block proposals that could erode industry profits by limiting drug prices or making it easier for people to buy low-cost generic versions of brand-name medicines. The industry was fighting legislation that would speed the approval and marketing of generic drugs.

WHO's evolving position

In May 2002, the World Health Assembly adopted a resolution 'Ensuring accessibility of essential medicines' (Res. WHA55.14). The resolution requested the Director-General, in part, to advocate the concept and policies of essential medicines as a tool for implementing rational prescription of medicines, to promote market-based differential pricing for essential medicines between high-, middle-, and low-income countries, and to provide technical support, especially to developing countries, to establish drug-pricing policies. WHO's medicine strategy was to address the important issue of the impact of international trade agreements on access to medicines. WHO should pursue all diplomatic and political opportunities aimed at overcoming barriers to access to essential medicines, in order to make them accessible and affordable to the people who need them. Finally, the Expert Committee on the Use of Essential Drugs should be strengthened in order to ensure its independence from external pressures at all times. The resolution identified the key issues: listing 'essential drugs' based on scientific evidence, ensuring drug quality and their rational use, ensuring equitable access to all drugs through, in particular, differential pricing. Showing the direct link between the drug industry and public health, it confirmed WHO's necessary, albeit reluctant at times, involvement in trade matters.

Currently, over one-third of the world's population lacks regular access to essential drugs (WHO, 2002e). In the poorest parts of Africa and Asia, this rises to over 50 percent. Education is needed in the rational use of drugs: up to 75 per cent of antibiotics are prescribed inappropriately, world wide, only 50 per cent of patients take their medicines correctly. On quality and safety, less than one in three developing countries has fully functioning drug regulatory authorities. Ten to 20 per cent of sampled drugs fail quality control tests in many developing countries. Failure in good manufacturing practices result, at times, in toxic or lethal products. For the 20 per cent of the global population who live in poverty, 60 per cent of deaths are due to diseases such as malaria and HIV/AIDS: many of those affected do not have access to effective treatment. Pharmaceutical expenditure in developing countries constitutes 25 to 65 per cent of total public and private health expenditure, and 60 to 90 per cent of out-of-pocket household spending on health (WHO, 2001f).

The WHO Constitution requires the Organization 'to develop, establish and promote international standards with respect to food, biological, pharmaceutical and similar products' (Art. 2 (u)). In September 1978, the Alma-Ata Conference convened jointly by WHO and UNICEF adopted the Strategy of 'Health for All by the Year 2000', based on the primary health care approach: one of its basic elements was the provision of essential drugs (Beigbeder, 1998: 21–29). The Conference recommended that Member States should:

> Formulate drug policies and regulations with respect to import, local production, sale and distribution of drugs and biologicals so as to ensure that essential drugs are available at the various levels of primary health care at the lowest feasible cost; that specific measures are taken to prevent the over-utilization of medicines; that proven traditional remedies are incorporated; and that effective administrative and supply systems be established (Koivusalo/Ollila, 1997: 163).

In 1969, WHO endorsed requirements for 'Good Practices in the Manufacture and Quality Control of Drugs'. In May 1978, the World Health Assembly urged Member States to enact legislation covering drug registration, use or prescription by generic names, control of drug information, price regulation (Res. WHA31.32). It requested the Director-General to develop further the dialogue with pharmaceutical industries, to study how prices of pharmaceutical products are determined and possible strategies for reducing such prices, including the development of a code of marketing practices, with special emphasis on pharmaceutical products essential for the populations of developing countries.

A new code of marketing practices could have been adopted by the Assembly as a regulation under Article 21 of the Constitution, or as a recommendation under Article 23, as the International Code of Marketing of Breast-milk Substitutes. Article 21 (e) gives authority to the Assembly to adopt regulations concerning 'advertising and labeling of biological, pharmaceutical and similar products moving in international commerce'. Through this resolution, the Assembly was intervening in the business practices of the pharmaceutical industry and potentially challenging its interests. After the adoption of the International Code of Marketing of Breast-milk Substitutes, it was proposing a second codification process.

However, the WHO Director-General, Dr. H. Mahler, after his unpleasant first experience of a conflictual codification process, chose to pursue consultations with the industry and avoid premature confrontations with the manufacturers and several Western countries. In 1985, a WHO conference of experts on the rational use of drugs was held in Nairobi. It was agreed that governments were responsible for regulating companies' marketing. The conference did not endorse the proposal for an international code on drugs. In 1986, the World Health Assembly approved a revised drug strategy based on the outcome of the Nairobi conference. Its policies, identified by WHO in 1988, had the following components:

- essential drugs lists, composed of a limited number of generic drugs;
- legislation, registration and quality assurance;
- procurement and distribution;
- local production;
- education and training;
- information to the public; and
- research (WHO, 1988).

During the World Health Assembly in 1986, the US re-asserted its position that WHO should not be involved in efforts to regulate and control the commercial practices of private industry, even when the products related to health. In 1986 and 1987, the US withheld its contribution to the budget of WHO, allegedly because of its disapproval of WHO's policies on breast food substitutes and essential drugs.

As from 1986, after having approved a revised drug strategy, the Assembly did not refer again to the formulation of a code of marketing practices. Through its resolutions, it supported the role of the Action Programme for Essential Drugs and WHO's support to countries in formulating, implementing and evaluating national drug policies and essential drug programmes. The implementation of the Programme was in effect being transferred from the international to the national level.

WHO Model List of essential drugs

In 1975, the World Health Assembly requested the Director-General to assist Member States by 'advising on the selection and procurement at reasonable cost, of essential drugs of established quality corresponding to their national health needs' (Res. WHA28.66). The first List was prepared by a WHO Expert Committee in 1977, and revised every two years thereafter (WHO, 2001g). By the end of 1999, 156 Member States had official essential drugs lists. The November 1999 Model List has 306 active ingredients, which include vaccines, contraceptives, preventive agents such as insect repellents and some diagnostic agents. The Model List is a guide for the development of national and institutional essential drug lists. It was not designed as a global standard. National lists usually relate closely to national guidelines for clinical health care practice for the training and supervision of health workers. They also guide the procurement and supply of drugs in the public sector, schemes that reimburse drugs costs, drugs donations, and local drug production. Many international organizations, including UNICEF and UNHCR, as well as NGOs and international non-profit supply agencies, have adopted the essential drug concept and base their drug supply system on the Model List.

Following a consultative process carried out in 2001, a revised procedure was approved for updating and disseminating the Model List. WHO agreed to use the term 'essential medicines' as an alternative to 'essential drugs', reflecting the common use of the term 'medicines' to describe pharmaceutical preparations used in clinical health practice. 'Essential medicines' were defined as those that satisfy the priority health care of the population. They are selected with due regard to disease prevalence, evidence on efficacy and safety, and comparative cost-effectiveness. Essential medicines are intended to be available within the context of functioning health systems at all times in adequate amounts, in the appropriate dosage forms, with assured quality, and at a price the individual and the community can afford. It was also agreed that the absolute cost of a medicine will not be a reason to exclude it from the Model List if it meets the selection criteria, and cost-effectiveness comparisons should be made among alternative medicines within the same therapeutic group.

The link with trade .

In May 1999, the World Health Assembly mandated the Director-General to monitor the public health consequences of international trade agreements, a mandate which was confirmed in May 2001 (Res. WHA52.19 and 54.11).

WHO was represented at the contested Conference of the World Trade Organization (WTO) held in Seattle from 30 November to 3 December 1999. WHO's intention was to ensure that trade and public health should not be discussed in isolation (WHO, 1999c). In particular, WHO said that it supported the incorporation, as stipulated in the Agreement on Trade-Related Aspects of Intellectual Property Rights (TRIPS), of patent protection into national legislation. WHO would collaborate with governments in applying the provisions of Article 66, which enables least developed countries to extend the transitional period for implementation of TRIPS. WHO also expressed support for the rapid production of generic products in order to promote competition and contain drug expenditure (the 'Bolar amendment'), – for drug prices consistent with local purchasing power, – for preferential pricing in poor countries. As a condemnation of the unfettered free market dogma, WHO expressed its concern with the 'obvious market failures that lead hundreds of millions of people being left without access to essential drugs'.

WTO and the TRIPS Agreement

As the legal and institutional foundation of the multilateral trading system, established in 1995, WTO promotes trade liberalization, the lowering of trade barriers, through the negotiation of multilateral agreements.

The TRIPS Agreement sets minimum standards of protection for intellectual property rights including patents, copyrights, trademarks and industrial designs, to be enforced through national legislation. The terms of protection for patents are set at a minimum of 20 years from the filing date. From 1 January 1995, the transitional periods agreed to upgrade their legal and regulatory systems to be compliant with TRIPS were one year for industrialized countries, five years for developing countries (until 2000), and at least eleven years (until 2006) for least developed countries.

During the term of a patent, the 'Bolar exception' in patent law permits research, development and submission of information and samples required of generic drug manufacturers by regulatory authorities for registration. Its purpose is to facilitate the approval of a a generic product for marketing before patent expiration, thereby permitting a prompt introduction of generic versions after that date, at a lower price than the patented medicines.

In theory, the Agreement allows countries to protect public health (Thomas, 2002: 254). Under Article 8.1, 'members may ... adopt measures necessary to protect public health and nutrition, and to promote the public interest in sectors of vital importance to their socio-economic and technological development'. Under certain circumstances, TRIPS allows countries to pursue parallel importing (Article 6, Exhaustion of Rights) and compulsory licensing (Article 31).

- Parallel imports refer to importing a patented drug from a third party in another country where it is sold for less. Under Article 28 of the TRIPS, patent owners have the right to prevent third parties from 'making, using, offering for sale, selling or importing' a product, but states determine when these rights are exhausted. Under Article 6, States can take whatever action they deem necessary at the point of exhaustion. This allows for parallel imports as national policy, permitted under EU, US and Japanese patent laws.
- Compulsory licensing permits the manufacture anywhere and use of generic drugs without the agreement of the patent holder. Under Article 31, States can issue such licenses for various reasons, not only national emergencies, so long as they adopt adequate safeguards such as compensation. In such emergencies, as in the case of non-commercial public use, or to correct anti-competitive practices, they do not need to make prior efforts to negotiate a licence on reasonable commercial terms with the patent holder.

A WHO/WTO Workshop on Pricing and Financing of Essential Drugs, held in Norway in April 2001 brought together a group of 80 experts from 21 countries and varied professional backgrounds. Strategic options suggested in the Workshop included creating the right conditions so that the market determines differential pricing, discounts negotiated bilaterally between companies and purchasers; licences agreed voluntarily between patent owners and generic manufacturers and global procurement and distribution systems. Critical to the success of differential pricing would be methods of preventing lower priced drugs from finding their way into rich markets (WHO, 2001h).

The Doha Ministerial Conference – 9–14 November 2001

In its final 'Declaration on the TRIPS Agreement and Public Health' adopted on 14 November 2001, the Conference recognized the gravity of the public health problems afflicting many developing and least-developed countries, while also recognizing the importance of intellectual property protection for the development of new medicines (WTO). The flexibility provided by the TRIPS Agreement gives the right to Members to grant compulsory licences and the freedom to determine the grounds upon which such licences are granted. Each Member has the right to determine what constitutes a national emergency or other circumstances of extreme urgency, it being understood that public health crises, including those relating to HIV/AIDS, tuberculosis, malaria and other epidemics, can be included in these terms. The Conference also agreed to provide an additional ten-year transition period (until 2016) for the least-developed Members with regard to pharmaceutical products.

During the negotiations, tensions rose between two groups: the US, supported by the European Union, Japan, Switzerland and Canada, and other developed countries, intent on preserving protection of intellectual property, and a coalition led by Brazil and India trying to strengthen health safeguards in the Agreement. The latter countries had placed their hopes on several recent events: the South African court victory in April 2001, – the passing of the Kenya Industrial Property Bill 2001 on 14 June 2001, which will allow Kenya to import and produce more affordable medicines for HIV/AIDS and other medicines, – in July 2001, the US withdrawal of its complaint against Brazil to WTO over Brazil's patent law and the transfer of the 'disagreement' to a newly created bilateral consultative mechanism (US, 2002a). In November 2001, during the anthrax crisis, the US Administration won a major price concession from the German drug company Bayer AG for its antibiotic ciprofloraxin (Cipro), after threatening to buy generic alternatives (Charatan, 2001). This showed that a pharmaceutical company could accept price reductions in case of a health emergency, and that the US did not hesitate to press for such a reduction, in spite of its stance as a staunch defender of patent rights and non-intervention in trade issues.

Dr Brundtland, the former WHO Director-General, said that she was pleased to hear of the Ministers' conclusions that the TRIPS Agreement 'can and should be interpreted and implemented in a manner supportive of WTO Members' right to protect public health and, in particular, promote access to medicines for all' (WHO, 2001i). Oxfam agreed and the NGO said that the Doha Declaration was an important step forward in the campaign for affordable medicines. 'It affirmed the primacy of public health over intellectual property rights, and the rights of governments to make full use of the public health safeguards in TRIPS' (Oxfam, 2002a).

Other observers were not so sure. The Declaration agreed that 'the TRIPS Agreement does not and should not prevent Members from taking measures to protect public health'. This statement, taken as a significant advance, was only a political statement, not a binding statement. There was no commitment to change the wording of the TRIPS Agreement to accommodate developing countries' overriding of patents for public health purposes, a victory for the North. NGOs present at the meeting deplored the 'high-handed unethical negotiating practices of the developed countries – linking aid budgets and trade preferences to the trade positions of developing countries and targeting individual developing country negotiators' (CorpWatch, 2001b; Bello, 2002).

The Report of the Commission on Macroeconomics and Health, published on 20 December 2001, gave support to the developing countries. It called for a new global framework for differential pricing of essential drugs for poorer nations. The group suggested that WHO, the pharmaceutical industry – patent holders and generic producers – and low income countries should work together to agree on guidelines. The Commission said that the TRIPS Agreement should be 'interpreted broadly' to ensure that poorer countries that cannot produce generic drugs can still get access to generic production from third countries. However, an IFPMA representative countered that the spotlight should not be on the drug industry but on governments of rich and poor nations (Ashraf, 2001).

After Doha

During the January 2002 meeting of the WHO Executive Board, the US representative openly expressed his profound disagreement with WHO's pursuit of 'certain goals' under the rubric of access to essential medicines, and with two documents submitted to the Board, Doc. EB109/7 and 109/8. (WHO, 2002f). He criticized certain sectors of the WHO Secretariat and WHO Membership as still having 'a profound bias against the private sector'. There was an inherent assumption that generic drugs were always preferable to those produced by the research-based pharmaceutical industry, an assumption that ignored quality control problems and the commercial interests of the generic drug sector. The US representative felt that Document EB109/7 (WHO, 2001f) had an overriding and inappropriate focus on drug pricing, cost-effectiveness and intellectual property questions, and a lack of focus on the normative functions of WHO. The TRIPS Agreement was not part of the problem of expanding drug access, but part of the solution. More than 95 percent of the drugs currently included in the WHO Model List of Essential Drugs were free of patent protection anywhere in the world, yet that had not increased access to most of these medicines in many nations. The US could not and would not support any effort to establish an international or multinational mechanism to regulate drug prices. It would continue efforts to provide market-based, voluntary ways of reducing prices across the world. Any attempt by WHO or other organizations to establish price guidelines or pricing schemes would be inappropriate. In April 2002, in its Annual 'Special 301' Report on Global Intellectual Property Protection, the Office of the US Trade Representative affirmed the US continued commitment to ensure effective intellectual property protection around the world (US, 2002b). 'US creativity and ingenuity improves the lives of people all over the world. American innovators, like our scientists, artists and writers, rely on intellectual property protection to safeguard their inventions and creations. Strong intellectual property protection should also be a priority for other countries because it will help them attract investment and technology'.

The Doha Declaration had recognized that WTO Members with insufficient or no manufacturing capacities in the pharmaceutical sector could face difficulties in making effective use of compulsory licensing under the TRIPS Agreement. It instructed the Council for TRIPS to find an expeditious solution to this problem and to report to the General Council before the end of 2002 (Article 6).

Delegates at the Council failed to reach an agreement by that deadline. MSF and Oxfam blamed the pharmaceutical industry, the US, Japan, the European Union and Switzerland for this failure (Oxfam, 2002b, – MSF, 2003a). These countries wanted to limit the number of diseases covered by the Agreement to HIV and AIDS, malaria, tuberculosis, or other infectious epidemics of comparable gravity and scale. Developing countries including Brazil, India and China contended that governments had the right to determine which diseases constituted public health crises in their countries. However, the rich countries, relaying the restrictive position of their pharmaceutical companies, feared that the list would be too large, possibly including such rich countries diseases as diabetes, hypertension and asthma. The US, which caused the breakdown of the negotiations, pledged that until a deal was reached, it would not initiate any complaint to the WTO for breaking the Agreement by exporting cheaper medicines to poor countries. The US urged other countries to join them in this moratorium (Becker, 2002).

In January 2003, Pascal Lamy (Lamy, 2003), the European Commissioner for trade, questioned the 'strident' concerns of the pharmaceutical industry that a compromise agreement had the potential to weaken research into new medicines as exaggerated. 'If the poor countries are unable in any case to buy the medicines, where are the lost profits for the industry, where is the problem?' Lamy's proposal was to involve WHO: countries would ask for guidance from WHO to assess the seriousness of public health problems. A WHO official replied that the national health authorities had the necessary competence to decide as to which were the emergencies (Benkimoun, 2003).

WTO members had aimed to establish by 31 March 2003 a framework for negotiations to reduce trade barriers and subsidies in agriculture: no agreement was reached by that date. Without agreement on agriculture, agreement on other trade issues would not be possible, as all areas of the negotiations are linked: there must be agreement on all issues. Another meeting of trade ministers was to take place in September 2003 in Cancun, Mexico and the Doha round is scheduled to be completed in January 2005. At the time of writing, the chances of an agreement by that date are uncertain.

Conclusion

Patent protection and the cost of medicines are two of several factors affecting poor people's access to medicines, and more generally, access to healthcare. Other factors include the country's political and economic position, its health policy, the budget share allocated to health, its health infrastructure, the supply of drugs, the capacity of its health personnel to administer medicines safely and efficaciously.

As intellectual property rights are being strengthened globally under the authority of WTO agreements and under the influence of the rich countries, the cost of medicines in developing countries is likely to increase, thus making the access to essential medicines more difficult for poor populations, unless effective steps are taken to facilitate their availability at lower cost in those countries, as noted by the Commission on Intellectual Property Rights.[2]

The Commission recognized that, without the incentive of patents, it is doubtful that the private sector would have invested so much in the discovery or development of medicines. 'But the evidence suggests that the IP [intellectual property] system hardly plays any role in stimulating research on diseases particularly prevalent in developing countries, except for those diseases where there is also a substantial market in the developed world (e.g. diabetes or heart disease)'.

Among the Commission's recommendations:

- Public funding for research on health problems in developing countries should be increased;
- The IP system can help to establish differential pricing mechanisms, which would allow prices for drugs to be lower in developing countries, while higher prices are maintained in developed countries;
- Developed countries should maintain and strengthen their legislation to prevent imports of low priced pharmaceutical products originating from developing countries;
- The legislation of developing countries should facilitate their ability to import patented medicines if they can get them cheaper elsewhere in the world (parallel imports);
- Developing countries should adopt legislation and procedures allowing them to use compulsory licensing;
- Developing countries should adopt legislation facilitating the entry of generic competitors as soon as the patent has expired on a particular drug, and avail themselves of the Bolar exception.

The pharmaceutical industry remains diffident towards such proposals. They fear the impact of generic drugs on their profits. They fear that patented drugs sold at lower prices in developing countries, or lower-priced generic drugs will be exported illegally to rich countries. It is however unlikely that patients in rich countries would buy and use illegal drugs without a clear indication of their origin and contents (formula). Health insurance schemes in those countries would not reimburse such purchases. Perhaps more basically, the industry fears that questions may be asked as to the legitimacy of the high prices of patented medicines, in relation to much lower prices of generic drugs. The pharmaceutical companies would rather not open this door widely: they agree to keep it only ajar, under strict control, i.e. to negotiate reduced prices case by case, country by country. They are still resisting a wider availability of generic drugs, as well as the production of generic drugs in developing countries.

Companies are required to obey national laws. In addition, those which have adhered to the UN Global Compact should act, in their corporate domains, on the principles drawn from the Universal Declaration of Human Rights, the ILO Labour Conventions and the Rio Principles on Environment and Development. As openly stated by a Novartis official, 'weaving universal values into the fabric of global markets and corporate practices would help advance broad social goals while securing open markets' (Leisinger, 2002). He submits that, for the pharmaceutical industry, there are two dimensions of their social responsibility. The 'ought to do' dimension includes flexibility for negotiated, differential pricing according to specific needs and demands, subject to several conditions to 'prevent an exploitation of goodwill': – control over trade to avoid re-exportation or leakage of the low-priced drugs to the markets of industrial countries, – an appropriate political environment, including a readiness on the part of consumers in high-priced markets to accept sustained price difference, – undertakings from industrial countries not to use differential prices intended only for poor countries as benchmarks for their own price regulation systems or policies.

Are these severe conditions, some of which are difficult to satisfy, serious, or are they mentioned only to show a good will of principle, and obstacles so high that they cannot be overcome?

The second 'ought to do' dimension is reasonable and should be met by most large companies without problems: the readiness to help out with donations in cases of acute emergency, as both a humanitarian gesture and an effective public relations exercise.

The 'can do' or desirable norms are dimensions of social responsibility which are neither required by law nor standard industry practice, i.e. corporate philanthropy. They include social, medical and training benefits to local employees and their families through subsidiaries situated in poor countries, donations of free products or free treatment as part of joint projects with international organizations. With limited costs, these actions give support to specific beneficial programmes, even if they are restricted to employees, and will enhance the good name of the firm.

The pharmaceutical industry is not the only actor in the area of access to medicines in developing countries. Governments of both industrialized and developing countries within their countries and, on a regional or global basis, as members of intergovernmental organizations are the decision makers as legislators of patent regulation and of the protection and welfare of their own populations.

However, the balance of power tilts squarely towards rich countries, the pharmaceutical industry and against poor countries. Voluntary action by the industry, whose main and natural concern is profit, will not suffice in giving more rights to patients.

Only continued strong pressures by NGOs and a more explicit support by WHO, UNICEF and other UN agencies are needed. WHO cannot remain neutral. In addition to its normative and scientific role, WHO should take a more 'activist' stance in supporting the 'health exception' in the WTO debates, and in helping developing countries to use the provisions of the TRIPS Agreement in the best interests of their nation's health. To this end, WHO needs the support of 'like-minded' countries in the North, developing countries and NGOs in order to maintain its policy in support of generic drugs, differential pricing, and to support exceptions to TRIPS. As suggested by Health Action International (2002), WHO should provide countries with examples or models of intellectual property legislation. As suggested by MSF (2002b), WHO should support across-the-border negotiations regarding the pricing of medicines for neighbouring countries with similar needs. The WHO secretariat should implement the World Health Assembly resolution of May 2002 (Res. 55.14): 'to pursue all diplomatic and political opportunities aimed at overcoming barriers to access to essential medicines'. The risk is for the

Organization to cause the displeasure of, and possible sanctions from, the USA and other North countries. However, WHO's business is not business but international public health.

Notes

1 According to *Le Monde* of 23 August 2001, a WHO official, G.V. (Colombian), Director of the Drug Action Programme was physically aggressed and threatened with death in May 2001 in Rio de Janeiro, then in Miami. He later received several anonymous telephone calls asking him to 'stop criticizing the pharmaceutical industry' and trying to deter him from attending a WTO meeting on intellectual property rights applicable to medicines. A complaint was filed and a judiciary investigation is proceeding. There is however no evidence of the link between these incidents and the pharmaceutical industry (see also *Libération*, 12 November 2001).

2 The Commission on Intellectual Property Rights was set up by the British government to look at how intellectual property rights might work better for poor people and developing countries. It first met in May 2001 under the chaimanship of Professor John Barton (USA) and its final report was published on 12 September 2002. The full text of the report is available on www.iprcommission.org.

Chapter 5

The Global HIV/AIDS Epidemic

The facts

According to the Joint UN Programme on HIV/AIDS (UNAIDS), by the end of 2001, 42 million people were living with HIV. By 2010, the world total may reach 60 to 100 million. In the absence of drastically expanded prevention and treatment efforts, 68 million people will die because of AIDS in the 45 most affected countries between 2000 and 2020, more than five times the 13 million deaths of the previous two decades of the epidemic in those countries (UNAIDS, 2002a).

At the end of 2001, 4.1 million people were already living with HIV/AIDS in South Asia. India, with 3.97 million people living with HIV, is second only to South Africa in the total number of people infected. In China, reported HIV infections rose nearly 70 per cent in the first six months of 2001, mostly through heterosexual contact. The Russian Federation and Eastern Europe are home to the fastest growing epidemic in the world.

In Botswana, the country with the highest HIV infection rates in the world, almost 39 per cent of all adults were living with HIV in 2002, up from less than 36 per cent in 2000. In six other African countries, the HIV prevalence rate in adults exceeds 20 per cent.

Worldwide, approximately half of all new adult infections are among young people aged 15–24. Almost 12 million young people are living with HIV, and about 6000 more become infected every day. Fourteen million children have lost one or both parents to AIDS. Less than four per cent of those in need in the developing world have access to anti-retroviral treatment.

Also globally, the incidence of HIV/AIDS among women is rising. In 1997, 41 per cent of HIV-infected adults were women. This rose to 49.8 per cent in 2001 (UNAIDS, 2002b).

The acquired immunodeficiency syndrome (AIDS) was first recognized in 1981 among homosexual men in the USA. The human immunodeficiency virus (HIV) – the virus that causes AIDS – was identified in 1983. Extensive spread of HIV appears to have begun in the late 1970s and early 1980s among men and women with multiple sexual partners in East and Central Africa and among homosexual and bisexual men in certain urban areas of the Americas, Western Europe, Australia and New Zealand. The virus has, since then, been transmitted to all continents and countries. Worldwide, 75 to 85 per cent of HIV infections in adults have been transmitted through unprotected sexual intercourse, with heterosexual intercourse accounting for more than 70 per cent. Infection is also transmitted through administration of infected blood or blood products or sharing of contaminated injection equipment, – or from an infected mother to her foetus or infant during pregnancy or delivery, or when breast-feeding.

In the absence of an effective, tested vaccine or effective cure for AIDS, the main tool for controlling the epidemics is through culturally sensitive information and education on how HIV is transmitted and how exposure to it can be minimized or eliminated. Desirable measures include HIV testing, the promotion of a safe sexual behaviour, in particular by the use of condoms, the provision of counselling, training of medical and other health personnel, education in schools. In the 1980s, drug therapies against AIDS have become available: AZT since 1987 – since 1996, combinations of anti-retroviral agents. They do not cure the disease but alleviate its symptoms and have prolonged the life of persons living with HIV and AIDS for substantial periods. However, the price of these treatments is beyond the reach of most patients in developing countries.

Denial, indifference, ignorance and other obstacles

In most countries, the growing expansion of the disease was denied on various grounds. It was first labelled as a disease of homosexuals, with limited impact on populations, and to be treated as a just punishment for the homosexuals' 'deviance and sins'. Heterosexual transmission was established in Africa in the 1980s through the research and efforts of such pioneers as Dr Peter Piot – now Executive Director of UNAIDS – , Dr Jonathan Mann, who initiated the WHO Global Programme on AIDS in 1987,[1] and others.

Western governments first showed indifference towards the spread of the disease, first believed to kill 'only' homosexuals and Africans. Despite early warnings, the West refused to confront the epidemic in the 1980s. Africans thought that this was an illness produced by the 'whites' to kill them. African and Asian public health officials and diplomats dismissed HIV and AIDS as problems for Europe and North America, not for them.[2] Soviet-era disinformation alleged that the CIA had concocted the virus for germ warfare. The USSR and satellite countries boasted that this was a typical bourgeois illness of the promiscuous capitalist world, which could not take root in their 'clean' political environments.

Initially, Western development assistance agencies did not engage in anti-AIDS campaigns in developing countries on the basis that there was no cure for the disease and that prevention and care would be too expensive.

Denial was a general reaction also in Asia. Chinese health officials only recognized in September 2002 that the epidemic was growing in their country by raising estimates of sufferers to one million – still a low estimate – and saying that China would start manufacturing a full complement of AIDS drugs if the Western pharmaceutical companies who hold the patents did not lower prices by the end of the year. China also applied for a $90 million grant from the Global Fund for AIDS, Tuberculosis and Malaria. However, at the same time, Chinese authorities had harassed, and finally detained Wan Yanhai, an outspoken AIDS activist (Rosenthal, 2002).

To avoid the stigma of 'having AIDS', many prefer ignorance. In Botswana, some 280,000 of its 1.6 million population are living with HIV. Life expectancy is set to decrease from over 64 in 1998 to 42 in 2010. Sixty six thousand children have lost their parents to AIDS (*The Economist*, 2002a). Under an AIDS control programme started in 2000, the Bill and Melinda Gates Foundation is contributing $50 million over five years, a contribution matched by Merck & Co, together with an unlimited supply of anti-retroviral medicines. However, the assurance of free treatment has, so far, failed to persuade most Bostwanans to get tested for HIV, or change their sexual behaviour, thus slowing the programme. The culture of denial still prevails (Grunwald, 2002).

Religious dogma, beliefs or practices have raised obstacles to effective prevention of HIV/AIDS. While the United Nations,[3] most governments and organizations involved in AIDS programmes have affirmed that condoms are the most realistic and effective ways to slow the spread of HIV, the Vatican has consistently opposed their use as twice sinful – both as contraceptives and as promoters of promiscuity. Its spokesmen also regularly question whether condoms prevent sexual transmission of the virus. In a meeting of the Southern Africa's Roman Catholic bishops held in July 2001 in Pretoria, they pronounced the 'widespread and indiscriminate promotion of condoms ... an immoral and misguided weapon in our battle against HIV-AIDS'. By undermining abstinence and marital fidelity they said 'condoms may even be one of the main reasons for the spread of HIV-AIDS' (de Young, 2001). The World Council of Churches, representing 342 Protestant and Orthodox Christian churches, is a supporter of all methods of prevention, including the use of condoms. Islam does not exclude condoms but condemns indiscriminate sexual activity, homosexuality and drug abuse (Ahya, 2002).

The denial by South Africa's President Thabo Mbeki that his country was facing a grave health crisis due to AIDS is an odd case of political obstinacy based at least in part on scientific ignorance, and in part on cultural grounds: its effect was to slow down the fight against AIDS in his country. Some five million of South Africa's 44 million people have HIV. Some seven million will have died of AIDS-related illnesses by 2010. Two hundred and fifty thousand already die from them every year. According to UNAIDS, the average life expectancy is only 47 years, instead of 66, because of AIDS. Mr Mbeki questioned figures about the size of the HIV/AIDS epidemic in South Africa and the link between HIV and AIDS. He argued that anti-AIDS drugs are too costly and may be more dangerous than AIDS itself. He refused to single out AIDS as a special threat, preferring to talk about general 'diseases of poverty'. He felt that publicity about AIDS cast a negative light on Africans and their alleged promiscuity (*The Economist*, 2002b). The South African government slowly emerged from denial through public pressures from former President Nelson Mandela and Archbishop Desmond Tutu, from the opposition movement Treatment Action Campaign (TAC), from its own population and from such NGOs as Médecins Sans Frontières and Oxfam. In December 2001, the Constitutional Court ordered the government to make nevirapine freely available to HIV-positive pregnant women at state facilities nationwide. In April 2002, the government finally agreed to offer AIDS drugs to all poor pregnant women infected with HIV to prevent the transmission of the virus to unborn babies. Drugs would also be offered for the first time in public hospitals (Swarns, 2002) to rape victims.

Initiatives by UN agencies

The WHO Global Programme on AIDS was created in 1987. In May, the World Health Assembly approved the Global AIDS Strategy built on three broad objectives: prevention of HIV infection, reduction of the personal and social impact of HIV infection, unifying national and international efforts against AIDS. WHO organized the first World AIDS day on 1 December of the same year.

The Joint United Nations Programme on HIV/AIDS (UNAIDS) was established in January 1996 in Geneva, as a co-sponsored programme bringing together UNICEF, UNDP, UNFPA, UNESCO, WHO and the World Bank, later joined by ILO. This creation was a response to criticisms expressed by a number of governments and other donors regarding the lack of coordination of actions carried out in the field by these organizations, occasional duplication of efforts and unnecessary rivalry. UNAIDS thus took over the lead responsibility previously assumed by WHO. As the principal advocate for worldwide action against HIV/ AIDS, the global mission of UNAIDS is to lead, strengthen and support an expanded response to the epidemic that will prevent the spread of HIV, provide care and support for those infected and affected by the disease, reduce the vulnerability of individuals and communities to HIV/AIDS and alleviate the socio-economic and human impact of the epidemic.

UNAIDS is a small organization with an annual budget of $60 million and a staff of 129 professionals. Its work is guided by a Programme Coordinating Board with representatives from 22 governments, from its seven cosponsors, and five representatives of NGOs, including associations of people living with HIV/AIDS, the first UN programme to include NGOs in its governing body. Initial laboratory partners were Glaxo Wellcome, F. Hoffman-La Roche and Virco N.V. In 1998, Bristol-Myers Squibb and Organon Teknika joined them.

Dr Peter Piot, Executive Director of UNAIDS, has promoted the association of the private sector in the fight against HIV/AIDS. Besides basic humanitarian concerns, he said that it was 'in the enlightened self-interest of any company that operates in a global economy, that sells its goods to overseas markets or imports goods from those markets, to take action now to reduce the spread of HIV'. The expected benefits for companies are reduced risks to important markets, customers and suppliers, enhanced corporate profile as a leader in the community, a reduced vulnerability to HIV/AIDS among workforces.

In 1997, the Global Business Council on HIV/AIDS was launched in Edinburgh with former President Nelson Mandela as its Honorary President. It includes major companies.[4] UNAIDS played a key role in its creation and works closely with it, although the Council is a separate, independent body (UNAIDS, 2001). UNAIDS also collaborates with The Prince of Wales Business Leaders Forum, the Conference Board, the World Economic Forum and Rotary International. The World Chambers Federation has joined forces with UNAIDS as an official partner of the 2002–2003 World AIDS campaign.

In May 2000, UNAIDS announced that a new dialogue had begun between five pharmaceutical companies – Boehringer Ingelheim, Bristol-Myers Squibb, Glaxo Wellcome, Merck & Co., and F. Hoffmann-La Roche – and UN organizations – UNAIDS, WHO, UNICEF and UNFPA – to explore ways to accelerate and improve the provision of HIV/AIDS-related care and treatment in developing countries. The companies were offering, individually, to improve significantly access to, and availability of, a range of medicines (UNAIDS, 2000b). In June, the Accelerating Access Contact Group was established to share information and to advise UNAIDS and its co-sponsors on accelerating access to HIV care, support and treatment.

Another meeting took place in April 2001 between the UN Secretary-General, Kofi Annan, Dr Brundtland, the WHO Director-General and Peter Piot, and a group of CEOs and senior executives of six companies – Abbott Laboratories, Boehringer Ingelheim, Bristol-Myers Squibb, GlaxoSmithKline, Hoffmann-La Roche, and Pfizer, to agree on further steps to be taken to improve access to better healthcare, HIV medicines and HIV-related medicines. Kofi Annan said that 'Encouraging the active participation of all partners in the fight against AIDS has become my personal priority'.

In a special session of the UN General Asssembly held from 25 to 27 June 2001, heads of State and of governments adopted a Declaration of Commitment on HIV/AIDS. It recognized that poverty, underdevelopment and illiteracy were among the principal contributing factors to the spread of HIV/AIDS. It noted that stigma, silence, discrimination and denial, and lack of confidentiality undermine prevention, care and treatment efforts. It stressed that gender equality and the empowerment of women are fundamental elements in the reduction of the vulnerability of girls and women to HIV/AIDS. It recognized that effective prevention, care and treatment strategies require behavioural changes and increased availability and non discriminatory access to, inter alia, vaccines, condoms, drugs, as well as increased research and development. There is a need to reduce the cost of drugs in collaboration with the private sector and pharmaceutical companies. Progress made in some countries is linked with strong political commitment and leadership at the highest levels (UN, 2001). It was however unfortunate that the top leaders of Asia, Eastern Europe and South America did not attend the special session.

In March 2002, WHO published the first list of HIV-related medicines which were found to meet WHO recommended standards, under the Access to Quality HIV/AIDS Drugs and Diagnostics project. The project is managed by WHO, but counts on the expertise of UNICEF, UNAIDS, UNFPA and the World Bank (UNAIDS, 2002c).

However, in May 2002, the Paris Chapter of the AIDS Coalition to Release Power (ACT UP Paris) released a statement condemning the Accelerating Access Initiative as 'a puppet of the pharmaceutical industry'. It said that after two years, the Initiative had only resulted in getting an additional 0.1 per cent of persons with AIDS into treatment (Baue, 2002).

In July 2002, WHO and the International AIDS Society launched new international guidelines for a public health response to the treatment of AIDS in resource-poor settings. For the first time, highly complex antiretroviral therapy was simplified so that it could be used in settings not having highly trained medical staff and sophisticated laboratories available to initiate and supervise treatment. The guidelines lower the technical barriers to HIV/AIDS treatment, thus broadening access to safe and practical treatment (WHO, 2002g).

In December 2002, the International HIV Treatment Coalition (ITAC) was launched by WHO, UNAIDS and more than 50 other institutions, including NGOs, governments, foundations, the private sector, academic and research institutions and international organizations. The Coalition will focus on information sharing, drug procurement, health care training, donor coordination and technical assistance to national HIV/AIDS treatment programmes (JOURN-AIDS, 2002).

Access to drugs

Free or low-cost drugs are not the whole solution to the epidemic: remedies include education, prevention, treatment, care, support, effective health services, research, under a strong government leadership. However, treatment in poor countries requires access to free or reasonably-priced drugs, and particularly to lower-priced generic drugs. It implies the national development of industrial capacity to produce generic drugs in various countries, and their commercialization. Countries without generic drug industry should be allowed to import generic drugs without sanctions.

Obstacles to cost reductions and the production and sale of generic drugs have been raised by pharmaceutical companies protecting their patents and governments protecting their companies. Cost reductions have been obtained in the last few years in a few countries which challenged WTO rules, by the producers of generic drugs in a few developing countries, with the support and encouragement of NGOs, which used effectively the media to mobilize international public opinion. WHO and UNAIDS have played a quieter supporting role.

A research study published by Oxfam in July 2002 on 'The case of anti-retrovirals in Uganda' showed that the availability of cheap generic medicines in developing countries plays a significant role in cutting the price of patented anti-retrovirals (ARVs) and in increasing the number of patients which have access to these medicines. Despite the fact that the big five pharmaceutical companies had agreed under the Accelerated Access Initiative to reduce the prices of ARVs, it was the introduction of generic equivalents from India in October 2000 that led to a significant fall in the price of the brand name medicines in Uganda (Oxfam, 2002c).

As noted in Chapter 4, 40 pharmaceutical companies dropped their case against the South African government in April 2001, thanks to an effective NGO campaign. The contested South African legislation allowed importation of affordable medicines and increased use of generic drugs.

The South African 'victory' was preceded, in February 2001, by the announcement made by the Indian generic drug manufacturer Cipla Ltd that it would sell its triple-combination therapy for AIDS to MSF for $350 per year per patient and to governments for $600 per year. The $350 price was a discount of 96 per cent off the price of the same combination in the US, which would cost about $10,400. In November 2000, Glaxo-Wellcome had threatened to sue Cipla when it tried to sell Duovir, its generic version of Glaxo's Combivir, in Ghana. Cipla had offered the drug for $1.74 a day; Glaxo had cut its price to $2, from $16. But even though the African regional patent authority said that Glaxo's patents were not valid in Ghana, Cipla backed down and stopped selling Duovir (McNeil, 2001). On 21 February 2001, GlaxoSmithKline (GSK) promised to supply charities with discounted drugs (BBC, 2001a). In November 2002, GSK said that it offered its full range of antiretrovirals at a not-for-profit preferential price to 63 of the world's poorest countries, including sub-Saharan countries. GSK had received regulatory approval from 11 countries to supply ARVs in special, tri-lingual 'Access' packs. It was expected that providing medicines in differentiated packaging would help prevent illegal diversion of preferentially-priced products (Global, 2002).

In March 2001, Merck said that it would make Crixivan available at $600 per patient per year – instead of $5000 in the US – and Stocrin, available for $500: both are taken in combination with other drugs as an HIV 'cocktail'. GlaxoSmithKline offered discounted drugs to employers and non-profit groups. Oxfam welcomes the move, but said that it did not address the central problem, the systematic use of patent rules to keep low-cost drugs out of poor countries (BBC, 2001).

In June of the same year, the US dropped its complaint against Brazil for allowing the production of generic AIDS-treatment drugs in that country. The US had filed a complaint with the WTO in February 2001 over a Brazilian law that permits a local company to manufacture a product, made by a foreign company, if that company fails to initiate production within three years. The US complained that this law was protectionist and discriminated against all imported products (BBC, 2001b). In 1994, Brazil's government urged domestic pharmaceutical firms to start manufacturing AIDS drugs. Because of Brazil's production, prices for AIDS drugs exclusively produced abroad have dropped nine per cent, but more than 70 per cent for those that compete with Brazilian generic brands. Because of the wide availability of generic drugs supported by $450 million in government funding for some 93,000 patients, AIDS deaths were cut in half between 1996 and 1999. The government spends about $4,500 per patient each year for typical drug treatment. In the US, similar treatment cost between $12,000 and $15,000 (Jones, 2001).

In January 2003, Pharmacia Corp. (acquired by Pfizer Inc.) announced at the World Economic Forum in Davos that it would allow generic drug companies to manufacture low-cost copies of its AIDS drug to sell in poor countries. Pharmacia will work with the International Dispensary Association in Amsterdam to provide licenses and technological skills to generic companies to make its drug Delavirdine, an anti-retroviral sold under the name Rescriptor. The plan is an alternative to compulsory licensing (CBS, 2003). In February, the Swiss firm Roche said that it had cut prices on its AIDS drugs to the least developed countries. It also agreed that it would not act against possible infringements on patents on AIDS drugs in those countries, and that it would not file for further patent protection on AIDS drugs in those countries in the future (*International Herald Tribune*, 14 February 2003).

Vaccine initiatives

Scientists agree that a preventive vaccine is the best hope for ending the epidemic. However, vaccine research and development commands only about 2 per cent of the $20 billion spent worldwide on AIDS prevention, research and treatment. Hence the need to stimulate efforts, at the international level, towards an effective HIV/AIDS vaccine. When WHO launched its Global Programme on AIDS in 1987, it was said that at least five years would be needed to develop a vaccine. In 2003, research is progressing, but a successful outcome is not yet in view.

In 1996, Dr. Seth Berkley created the International AIDS Vaccine Initiative (IAVI), a global organization working to speed the research, development and distribution of preventive AIDS vaccines: 1996 was the year when UNAIDS was set up. Its work focuses on four areas: mobilizing support through advocacy and education, accelerating scientific progress, encouraging industrial participation in AIDS vaccine research and development, and assuring global access. IAVI has negotiated intellectual property agreements with its industry partners to help ensure that the future vaccine will be readily available in developing countries at reasonable prices. IAVI's partners are the World Bank, policy makers and industry leaders. It works with governments to promote the creation of national AIDS vaccine programmes. It also works with scientists and members of AIDS-affected communities. Foundations (Gates, Rockefeller, Lévi-Strauss, Starr, Sloan) have made donations to IAVI. IAVI has designed the *Scientific Blueprint for AIDS Vaccine Development.*

IAVI has created AIDS Vaccine Development Partnerships which bring together research, development, manufacturing and clinical trial expertise from both industrialized and developing countries with the goal of designing and developing AIDS vaccines specifically targeted for use in countries hardest hit by HIV and AIDS. It has laid the foundation for national AIDS vaccine programmes in South Africa, India and China.

IAVI has been associated with vaccine tests in Thailand and Uganda. In 1991, WHO designated Thailand as a country ready to test AIDS vaccines. With the support of UNAIDS, efficacy trials were conducted in Thailand with 2,500 injecting drug users, and in the USA, mostly gay white men. In February 2003, VaxGen, a company based in California, announced that there was no significant difference in protection between the 3,300 participants who received its vaccine, AIDSVax, and the 1,700 patients who got a placebo (Gellene, 2003). Trials of another series of preventive AIDS vaccines started in Uganda in February 2003, also with the support of IAVI (IAVI, 2003).

In February 2000, WHO and UNAIDS announced the creation of their HIV Vaccine Initiative to promote the development of a vaccine. In 1991, WHO spearheaded a vaccine development effort that assisted Brazil, Thailand and Uganda in elaborating the framework to conduct vaccine trials under the highest ethical and scientific standards. UNAIDS is bringing to the Initiative its expertise in social and behavioural research and community participation, which is essential to the conduct of human vaccine trials. WHO brings its vast experience in vaccinology and the conduits it has established with pharmaceutical firms in developing earlier vaccines. WHO would play an essential role in the delivery of an effective vaccine, when discovered (WHO/UNAIDS, 2000).

International financing

Aware that the limited financial resources of developing countries would delay or even block any progress in fighting the HIV/AIDS epidemic, Kofi Annan, the UN Secretary-General, launched the idea of a global AIDS and health fund in Abuja in April 2001. The economist Jeffrey Sachs had previously estimated that it would take about $10 billion annually to mount extensive but feasible prevention and treatment programmes in poor and middle-income countries. In May 2001, Annan told the World Health Assembly that 'the devastation wrought by HIV/AIDS is now so acute that it has itself become one of the main obstacles to development'. He said that plans were under way for the creation of an international fund to combat HIV/AIDS, tuberculosis and malaria, as a major tool for economic growth in the developing world (UNAIDS/WHO, 2001).

At the urging of Annan and national leaders, the UN General Assembly Special Session on HIV/AIDS, held in June 2001, supported the establishment of a global HIV/AIDS and health fund. From $7 to 10 billion was set as an expenditure target for the fight against the epidemic by 2005. In July 2001, the G8 leaders meeting in Genoa committed $1.3 billion to the fund.

The Global Fund to Fight AIDS, Tuberculosis and Malaria was set up in Geneva as an independent, public-private partnership working to attract, manage and disburse new resources to fight these diseases, and to rapidly disburse these funds to effective prevention and treatment programmes in countries in greatest need. The Fund is governed by a Board consisting of 14 government representatives, two NGO representatives and two private sector representatives. UNAIDS, WHO and the World Bank hold non-voting seats on the Board.

In April 2002, Dr Richard Feachem was named Executive Director of the Fund's board. The first call for projects resulted in more than 300 proposals. At the same meeting, the Fund awarded a total of $378 million over two years to 40 programmes in 3 countries, in addition to 18 proposals selected for a fast-track process. By July 2002, just over $1.9 billion in pledges to the Fund had been confirmed, mainly from the public sector (Global Fund, 2002).

Financial support has so far been disappointing. In July 2002, Oxfam said that rich countries must urgently give more money to the Fund if it is to have any impact on tackling the HIV/AIDS crisis. 'The response of donors to date is appalling. The $10 billion a year needed to combat AIDS is equivalent to just four days global military spending or what rich countries spend on agricultural subsidies in ten days' (Oxfam, 2002d). Private sector support has also been limited, except for a $100 million pledge by the Gates Foundation. At the World Economic Forum held on 6–7 December 2001, the Fund held a consultation meeting with representatives of more than 20 multinational companies and international business federations, half of which were from the pharmaceutical industry. The participants endorsed the partnership but expressed 'significant concern that it will not succeed unless the private sector is fully recognized as a partner – not just as a potential donor'. The representatives wanted greater private sector involvement in all stages of the funding process, including technical review. The fact that there were only two private sector representatives – one from the Gates Foundation and one from McKinsey & Co – 'was seen as too little to credibly demonstrate a commitment to full parnership with the private sector' (Ramsay, 2002).

NGOs – Health Action International, the Health Gap Coalition, ACT UP Paris and Oxfam UK – had a different view: the Fund should have consumer representation, not industry representation. The voices of people with AIDS, as well as other consumers, must determine the priorities of the Fund. Representation from commercial interests in any governing or advisory capacity must be forbidden.

Money for purchase of treatment must be maximized through bulk procurement mechanisms, and the inclusion of generic drugs (HAI, 2001).

On 28 January 2003, President George W. Bush announced, during his State of the Union speech, that his administration would ask the US Congress to approve an additional $10 billion to combat the AIDS epidemic in Africa. If approved, this would bring the total US commitment to $15 billion over five years. The President said that the initiative would provide enough funding to provide anti-AIDS drugs to two million people, mostly in Southern Africa, and provide medical care to 10 million people with AIDS and orphaned children, as well as AIDS prevention education programmes. The $15 billion virtually triples the current US commitment to fighting AIDS internationally. It includes $10 billion in new funds, of which $1 billion is for the Global Fund to Fight HIV/AIDS, Tuberculosis and Malaria (Baker, 2003).

The announcement was warmly received by officials of Southern African countries and some NGOs, hoping that other wealthy countries would follow suit. Other NGOs felt that the US should contribute at least $2.5 billion a year to the Global Fund. The executive director of the Global AIDS Alliance found Bush's pledge encouraging, but wrote that only five percent of the new spending was requested in the President's budget. This budget cut nearly in half the level of financing authorized by Congress for the Global Fund. To finance the proposal, the budget also proposed cuts in children's health programme (Zeitz, 2003).

In July 2003, President Bush named a former pharmaceutical company executive to coordinate the administration's global AIDS policy, Randall Tobias, the former chairman and chief executive of Eli Lilly & Co.

Conclusion

The spread of the AIDS epidemic will require more and more funds over the next few years. UNAIDS estimates that $10.5 billion will be needed in 2005 for prevention, care and support programmes in low and middle income countries – by 2007, some $15 billion will be required. Substantial increases in expenditures should be provided from all quarters – governments, bilateral and multilateral agencies, NGOs and the private sector. Most of the funds should come from increased development assistance as well as debt relief. The creation of the Global Fund to fight AIDS, Tuberculosis and Malaria is a positive initiative, but it remains underfunded. It is unfortunate that the Fund, which was initially designed to fight AIDS only, had its mandate expanded to two other diseases, thus blurring its scope and decreasing its power of attraction. All current expenditures and pledges to fund AIDS programmes, at the national and international levels, are still inadequate. Further mobilization should be stimulated by WHO and NGOs.

The reduction of prices of patent medicines and generics, through increased national production of generic drugs and pressures by NGOs plays a significant role in limiting expenses. Price reduction also increases the availability of effective treatment to people with HIV/AIDS in developing countries.

Dr Brundtland said in 2001 that 'Popular outrage, political will, market forces, and the best science are enabling the pursuit of a fundamental principle of public health: the supply of essential medicines on the basis of need rather than on the ability to pay' (WHO, 2001j). WHO has taken position in favour of differential pricing subject to respecting patents' rights: mechanisms were needed to prevent illicit re-export of lower priced drugs into richer economies.

Both WHO and UNAIDS recognize the necessity of working with pharmaceutical companies, and not against them. They are the main source of research and development of new medicines and other medical products, besides the less funded non-commercial laboratories. They are to be convinced that their own self-interest is to work with, and not against, the international organizations concerned with public health. However, IGO's rhetoric about the health needs of poor countries cannot achieve what NGOs have achieved through strong and vocal campaigns, and threats of boycott.

As from 2001, governments of a few developing countries, aware of the dramatic consequences of the HIV/AIDS epidemic and prepared to face threats and sanctions from Western countries, have won their first battles against the major pharmaceutical companies, with the effective backing of NGOs.

WHO is in a dilemma: should it support these governments and NGOs at the risk of antagonizing its main funding contributors, or should it remain 'neutral'. But WHO cannot remain neutral: its mandate demands that it facilitate equity access of effective medicines to poor countries. Effective price reductions of AIDS drugs have been obtained by pressures from NGOs, not by WHO. WHO has not forcefully supported the production of generic drugs by developing countries. NGOs have done so. More battles will have to be fought, not only by NGOs but also by a more outspoken WHO, in the forthcoming WTO negotiations before the transition period set by the TRIPS Agreement comes to an end on 1 January 2016.

Notes

1 Dr Mann died in a plane accident on 3 September 1998. He had left WHO in 1990 after disagreements with the WHO Director-General, Dr. Hiroshi Nakajima.
2 See W.W. Furth's Letter to the Editor, 'AIDS in Africa was no secret', *International Herald Tribune*, 12 July 2000.
3 See for instance the Declaration of Commitment on HIV/AIDS of 27 June 2001, para. 23, UN Doc. A/s-26/L.2.
4 Among them: Bristol-Myers Squibb, Calvin Klein, Cargill, Edelman Communications, GlaxoSmithKline, Merck & Co. In 2001, The Coca-Cola Company, Unilever, Viacom and AOL Time Warner joined the Council. Richard Holbrooke is its current President and CEO.

PART III
PUBLIC-PRIVATE PARTNERSHIPS
FOR HEALTH

Chapter 6

Controlling Onchocerciasis

The Onchocerciasis Control Programme (OCP), launched in 1974 by the World Bank in association with WHO and other partners, is considered a pioneer and successsful model of public-private partnerships for health.

A public-private partnership on neglected health problems is a combination of various skills and resources in institutions from the public and private sectors aimed at effectively tackling health problems which persist in the face of independent action, in particular those diseases that disproportionately affect the poor in developing countries.[1] In traditional health collaborations, associate organizations maintain autonomous decision-making to fulfil their individual objectives and contribute mainly by providing financing which covers the costs of the activities. In the new models of collaboration between public and private sectors, partners engage in shared decision-making to reach a shared objective. Additionally, they may provide resources and skills that the other institutions lack. OCP has associated the World Bank, WHO, UNDP and FAO, donor countries and agencies, NGOs and a business partner, Merck & Co., which has donated unlimited doses of its medicine, Mectizan®. The World Bank has provided leadership and funding, WHO, technical expertise and operational management.

The disease and its impact

Onchocerciasis is the world's second leading infectious cause of blindness, and is present in 35 countries of Africa, the Arabian peninsula and the Americas. Out of some 120 million people worldwide who are at risk of the disease, 96 per cent are in Africa. Of the 35 countries where the disease is endemic, 28 are in sub-Saharan Africa, six are in the Americas, and one is in the Middle East. A total of 18 million people are infected with the disease and have dermal microfilariae, of whom 99 per cent are in Africa. Of those infected with the disease, over 6.5 million suffer from severe itching or dermatitis and 270,000 are blind (WHO, 2000b).

Onchocersiasis is caused by *Onchocerca volvulus*, a parasitic worm that lives for up to 14 years in the human body. Each adult female worm produces millions of microscopic larvae that migrate throughout the body and give rise to a variety of symptoms. Serious visual impairment, including blindness, rashes, lesions, intense itching and depigmentation of the skin, lymphadenitis, which results in hanging groins and elephantiasis of the genitals and general debilitation. Onchocerciasis manifestations begin to occur in persons one to three years after the injection of infective larvae. Microfilariae produced in one person are carried to another by the blackfly, which in West Africa belongs to the *Simulium damnosum* species complex. The blackfly lays its eggs in the water of fast-flowing rivers. Adults emerge after 8–

12 days and live for up to four weeks, during which they can cover hundreds of kilometres in flight. After mating, the female blackfly seeks a bloodmeal and may ingest microfilariae if the meal is taken from a person infected with onchocerciasis. A few of these microfilariae may transform into infective larvae within the blackfly, which are then injected into the person from whom the next meal is taken and subsequently develop into adult parasites, thus completing the life cycle of the parasite.

Apart from its health impact, onchocerciasis has an important socio-economic impact in view of the crippling effect of the disease causing a loss of productivity. Another negative impact is the forced migration of communities from the areas where the flies breed, the fast flowing rivers, often the most fertile land.

The three programmes

Two programmes in Africa and one in the Americas have been developed to fight against onchocerciasis.

The Onchocerciasis Control Programme (OCP)

In 1972, scientists discovered a way to combat onchocerciasis with aerial spraying, which destroyed blackfly larvae. Convinced of the potential effectiveness of this method, Robert McNamara, then World Bank president, organized an international effort to finance the future Onchocerciasis Control Programme (OCP). The programme was the first large-scale health effort initiated by the World Bank.

OCP was launched in 1974 in an area which originally included seven countries in West Africa, then extended in 1986 to four additional countries.[2] The total operational area covers 1.23 million sq. km and a combined population of about 30 million persons.

OCP's initial method for controlling onchocerciasis has been to break the cycle of transmission by eliminating the black fly. Simulium larvae are destroyed by application of selected insecticides through aerial spraying of breeding sites in fast-flowing rivers. Once the cycle of river blindness has been interrupted for 14 years, the reservoir of adult worms dies out in the human population, thus eliminating the source of the disease. As from 1989, vector control was complemented by therapeutic treatment. OCP then distributed Mectizan (ivermectin) through a community directed approach. Mectizan kills the larval worms that cause blindness and other onchocercal manifestations and acts to decrease transmission as well.

OCP ended in 2002, as well as its strategy of aerial larviciding. Aerial spraying of larvicide blanketed an area of 1.3 million square kilometers, in which 30 million people lived. At its launch, more than one million people in West Africa suffered from the disease, of whom 100,000 had serious eye problems including 35,000 people who were blind. At the end of the programme, the number of infected people within the area of operations is practically nil. Some 1.5 million people who were once infected with onchocerciasis no longer have any trace of the disease. Eleven million children born in the operational area since the programme's inception are free of risk of contracting the disease. By the end of 1999, it was estimated that OCP had prevented almost 300,000 cases of blindness in the 11 countries of the programme.

The successful onchocerciasis vector control activities have opened up an estimated 25 million hectares of fertile riverine land for resettlement and cultivation, land which was previously deserted for fear of the disease. This land has the potential to feed an additional 17 million people annually through the use of indigeneous technologies and farming practices.

OCP has been jointly sponsored by the World Bank, WHO, UNDP and FAO, and was supported by a coalition of more than 20 donor countries and agencies. WHO has acted as the executive agency for the programme, while the World Bank was responsible for mobilizing resources and administering the OCP Trust Fund. The estimated total cost for the programme was $550 million, or less than $1 per year for each protected person.

In 2003, the 11 participating countries have taken over the responsibility of carrying out the residual activities of monitoring and controlling the disease, including the distribution of Mectizan.

The African Programme for Onchocerciasis Control (APOC)

Building on OCP's success, APOC was launched in 1995. It shares the same co-sponsoring agencies and donors as OCP. Its objective is to establish, within a period of 12 years, sustainable community-directed ivermectin distribution systems covering about 50 million people in 17 countries outside OCP where onchocerciasis is still a serious public health problem.[3] In these countries, it is estimated that of the 15 million heavily infected people, 6.4 million live in areas where the parasite strains are a major cause of blindness while 8.6 million live in areas where the parasite strains are responsible for severe skin disease associated with grave and unrelenting itching. The principal control strategy, ivermectin treatment is complemented with vector elimination using environmentally safe methods.

Since its inception, APOC management has been set up at the OCP headquarters in Ouagadougou (Burkina Faso) and National Onchocerciasis Task Forces have been created in 14 countries. APOC's goal is to treat about 45 million people by 2007.

In 1996, the Non-Governmental Development Organizations (NGDOs) Coordination Group for Onchocerciasis Control facilitated distribution to 7.5 million people, This number increased to 11.7 million in the first year of APOC's field activities (1997–1998) and rose to over 15 million by the end of 1999.

In December 2001, the Annual Meeting of APOC and OCP announced that $39 million had been pledged to eliminate the disease in the whole of Africa by 2010. The new funds, to be complemented over the next few years to reach a total of $80 million, will bring the figure of people treated up to 60 million per year by 2010 (World Bank, 2002).

The Onchocerciasis Elimination Program in the Americas (OEPA)

Following the free donation of Mectizan by Merck & Co. in 1987, efforts to mass distribute the drug came from NGDOs which had, by 1989, already established projects in Africa and Latin America. In the Americas, the Pan American Health Organization (PAHO), also serving as WHO's Regional Office for the Americas, called for the elimination of all morbidity from onchocersiasis from the region by the year 2007 through mass distribution of ivermectin. Since 1991, a multinational, multi agency partnership has been assembled, composed of PAHO, the endemic countries,[4] NGDOs, the US Centers for Disease Control and Prevention in Atlanta, Georgia, as well as academic institutions and funding agencies. This partnership is embodied in the OEPA, which was supported by the River Blindness Foundation and by the Carter Center (Blanks, 1998).

Merck's donation

In 1987, Merck & Co., Inc. announced the donation free of charge for as long as necessary, wherever needed, to help bring the onchocerciasis under control as a public health problem.[5] In 1987, the Mectizan Donation Program was launched to oversee the donation and ensure that the drug was distributed in accordance with good medical practice. In 1998, Merck announced the extension of the programme to include the donation of Mectizan for the control of lymphatic filariasis in African countries where onchocerciasis and filariasis co-exist.

As reported by Merck, the power of Mectizan is its ability, with just one annual dose, to paralyze the microscopic worms that cause the effects of onchocerciasis. Without the worms' constant movements, itching stops and blindness can be avoided. Although the medicine does not kill the adult worms, it prevents them from producing additional offspring for up to 12 months, when the person is scheduled to receive his or her next annual dose. Mectizan requires little after-treatment monitoring in patients. It also has few dietary or storage requirements, making treatment possible in the most remote areas, far from health care facilities.

Research by a Merck veterinary scientist and an interdisciplinary team showed in the 1970s showed that ivermectin was extremely effective against parasites in many animals. In 1982, Merck and WHO began a collaborative ivermectin research programme in people. Clinical trials were carried out in West African countries which showed the effectiveness and ease of administering Mectizan. The seven-year trial process led to the clearance of Mectizan by French regulatory authorities in 1987.

Internal debates then followed at Merck. What price, if any, should the company charge for Mectizan? The company's quandary was that the people who could benefit from this medicine were also the least able to pay for it. If the company donated the medicine, would it create an expectation that future medicines for diseases in the developing world would be donated? Would this philanthropic act prove, in the long run, to be a disincentive for research against tropical diseases? In addition to manufacturing and administrative costs, what risks would Merck face if Mectizan caused unexpected adverse reactions? (Merck, 2003).

The final decision, taken in October 1987, was free donation of Mectizan for the treatment of river blindness to all who need it for as long as needed.

In 1988, Merck announced the formation of the Mectizan Expert Committee (MEC), an independent group of experts in tropical medicine and public health. The

Committee reviews and approves applications from NGDOs, ministries of health and local health agencies for free supplies of the medicine. Applicants have to demonstrate the ability to deliver Mectizan effectively for at least five years, to report serious adverse experiences and to keep accurate records. Also in 1988, Merck established the Merck Mectizan Donation Program (MDP), as part of the Task Force for Child Survival & Development, an affiliate of Emory University.[6] The MDP maintains liaison with Merck and WHO and is headquartered in Atlanta, Georgia. The Carter Center, through its Global 2000 River Blindness program (GRBP), is one of the more than 70 organizations involved in the programme. It assists ministries of health in ten countries to distribute ivermectin The GRBP's priorities are to maximize ivermectin treatment coverage and related health education and training efforts, and to monitor progress through regular reporting of ivermectin treatments measured against annual treatment objectives and ultimate treatment goals, e.g. full coverage, defined as reaching all persons residing in at risk villages who are eligible for treatment (Richards, 2001).

Merck explains its philanthropic gesture by linking it to its credo and tradition. In the 1940s, streptomycin was the first antibiotic to be effective against tuberculosis. Merck owned exclusive rights to the drug. George W. Merck, the company's head from 1925 to 1950, and son of its founder, released its hold on the patent, thus allowing any company to manufacture streptomycin and effectively keeping its cost minimal and hundreds of people alive. After World War II, Merck sold the drug at cost to Japan. In a 1950 address at the Medical College of Virginia, in a mixture of altruistic service to patients and realistic need for profits, George W. Merck said: 'Medicine is for the people. It is not for the profits. The profits follow, and if we have remembered that, they have never failed to appear'. Merck's current mission statement includes: 'Our business is preserving and improving human life ... We value above all our ability to serve everyone who can benefit from the appropriate use of our products and services, thereby providing lasting consumer satisfaction' (Backus and Cabral, 2001).

Conclusion

The success story of the onchocerciasis programmes is due to a large extent to the discovery that ivermectin is an effective treatment against the disease. If a similar medicine had been found to combat malaria, no doubt the long and, so far, unsuccessful, battles against this disease would have followed the path opened by the onchocerciasis programmes. It is a success story, compounded by Merck's free donation of the medicine for as long as needed, and possibly a model for other public-private health partnerships.

Merck's donation is a philanthropic gesture which contributes effectively to the programmes, otherwise financed by the World Bank and carried out under the aegis of WHO, with operational assistance by many NGOs. It adds resources to a vertical programme targeting a specific disease in endemic countries, thus benefitting the programmes. Merck could have chosen other alternatives: offer Mectizan to WHO, the World Bank and affected countries at reduced cost, or at cost, rather than a totally free supply. The benefits for Merck are the promotion of its image as an enterprise concerned with a disease affecting poor populations in poor countries, a useful public relations exercise, particularly when 'big pharma' is under attack. However, to Merck's credit, the free donation was decided upon in 1987, well before the South African débacle of April 2001 and NGO campaigns against the pharmaceutical industry which were mostly started also in 2001. Another benefit is to show Merck's proximity and cooperation with WHO in a successful programme.

By the end of 2002, the value of Merck's donation of Mectizan® tablets was approximately $1,275,000,000,[7] to which are added about $250,000 per year for shipping costs and $1 to 1.5 million in administrative costs for the Mectizan Expert Committee and daily programme operations in Atlanta. These costs are not insignificant, even if related to Merck's consolidated net income for 2002 of $7,149.5 million, and $51.8 billion of consolidated sales for the same year (Merck, 2002). Even if its donation provides the firm with a tax reduction benefit, it is a voluntary, generous and useful contribution to this particular international public health programme.

The onchocerciasis programmes are carried out with the approval of WHO, the executing agency for the African programmes, and with the approval and full involvement of national ministries of health. Merck's donation is not in conflict with WHO Guidelines for Drug Donations, revised in 1999 (WHO, 1999d). The aim of the Guidelines is to improve the quality of drug donations, not to hinder them. They are not an international regulation, but are intended to serve as a basis for national or institutional guidelines. The Guidelines were mostly a response to problems experienced in emergency situations, but they are also relevant to corporate donations in non-emergency situations. The core principles of the Guidelines are as follows:

- a drug donation should benefit the recipient to the maximum extent possible;
- all donations should be based on an expressed need and unsolicited drug donations are to be discouraged;
- a donation should be made with full respect for the wishes and authority of the recipient and be supportive of existing government health policies and administrative arrangements;
- there should be no double standards in quality;
- donations should be based on an expressed need and should not be sent unannounced.

None of these principles has been breached by the Merck donations.

In contrast with other public-private partnerships, the onchocerciasis partnerships have not been opposed or criticized by NGOs or other observers. The implementation of this particular partnership has escaped the usual criticisms about the dangers of a close association of a public health organization with a profit-making enterprise: it appears that both parties, and more importantly the afflicted people, have benefited from these programmes.

Notes

1 A definition given by the Geneva Initiative on Public-Private Partnerships for Health.
2 The initial countries were Benin, Burkina Faso, Ghana, Côte d'Ivoire, Mali, Niger and Togo. Then Guinea, Guinea-Bissau, Senegal and Sierra Leone joined the programme. OCP headquarters was in Ouagadougou, Burkina Faso.
3 Angola, Burundi, Cameroon, Chad, the Central African Republic, the Congo, the Democratic Republic of the Congo, Ethiopia, Equatorial-Guinea, Gabon, Liberia, Malawi, Mozambique, Nigeria, Uganda, Sudan and Tanzania.
4 Brazil, Colombia, Ecuador, Guatemala, Mexico and Venezuela.
5 The main facts in this section are based on information issued by Merck's 'The Story of Mectizan, 2003 and by Mectizan Donation Program, The Task Force for Child Survival and Development, 2001, plus information given on 17 April 2003 by Merck officials. Assessment in the Conclusion is by the authors.
6 Among the NGDOs affiliated with the Merck Mectizan Donation Program: Lions Club International, Médecins Sans Frontières, OXFAM, Rotary International, World Vision International.
7 For approximately 850,000,000 tablets at $1.50 per tablet. Information on tablet value and costs was also given by Merck officials on 17 April 2003. Not included is the cost of various staff in the Office of Contributions, Manufacturing and Finance at Merck's headquarters in New Jersey who spend time on the programme.

Chapter 7

The Eradication of Poliomyelitis

The Global Polio Eradication Initiative is another example of an international public-private partnership targeting a single disease with substantial success. Instead of an effective treatment, as in the case of the onchocerciasis programmes, the programme provides an effective protection through a vaccine which prevents polio infection. The polio coalition includes IGOs, governments, NGOs, corporate partners and foundations, with the all-important role of Rotary International[1] in funding, social mobilization of communities and volunteers, and implementation of operations. As in the onchocerciasis case, it appears that the public-private association has proved beneficial to all concerned parties.

The disease and its impact

Poliomyelitis (polio) is a highly infectious disease caused by one of three related enteroviruses (WHO, 1997a). The virus usually enters the body through the mouth and then multiplies inside the throat and intestines. The incubation period is 4–35 days and the initial symptoms include fever, fatigue, headache, vomiting, constipation (or less commonly diarrhoea), stiffness in the neck and pain in the limbs.

Once established, poliovirus can enter the bloodstream and invade the central system – spreading along nerve fibres. As it multiplies, the virus destroys the motor neurons which activate muscles. These nerves cannot be regenerated and the affected muscles no longer function. Muscle pain, spasms, and fever are associated with the rapid onset of acute flaccid (floppy) paralysis.

Polio paralysis is almost always irreversible. The muscles of the legs are affected more often than the arm muscles. More extensive paralysis, involving the trunk and muscles of the thorax and abdomen, can result in quadriplegia. One in 200 infections leads to irreversible paralysis (usually in the legs). Among the paralysed patients, five to ten per cent die when their breathing muscles become immobilized. The disease can strike at any age but polio affects mainly children under three years of age (50–70 per cent of all cases). As there is no cure for polio, the best (and only) treatment is preventive. A few drops of the oral polio vaccine (OPV), given multiple times, protects a child for life.

The eradication of polio

Polio eradication is technically feasible because there is no natural animal reservoir or long-term carrier state of poliovirus, and the virus cannot easily persist in tropical environments. In addition, there is an effective, low-cost, oral polio vaccine that provides intestinal and humoral immunity, and can interrupt circulation of the virus. However, according to WHO specialists (Birmingham *et al,* 1996), polio eradication faces two medical challenges. First, there is a high inapparent infection rate: less than one per cent of poliovirus infections result in paralysis. Secondly, this paralysis may be clinically indistinguishable from other conditions, notably infection with enterovirus 71 and Guillain-Barre Syndrome. These factors make laboratory confirmation by virus isolation necessary for definitive diagnosis of polio.

The Global Polio Eradication Initiative

In 1988, the Forty-first World Health Assembly launched a global initiative to eradicate polio by the end of the year 2000. This resolution (WHA41.28) followed the successful eradication of smallpox in 1979, and it was prompted by the progress made towards polio eradication in the Western Hemisphere. It was also encouraged by Rotary International's creation of its 'Polio-Plus' programme in 1985. In the same year, the Pan American Health Organization (PAHO) adopted a resolution to eradicate polio from the Americas by 1990. By 1991, the last clinical case of polio was reported from the region, and the Americas were certified as polio-free by 1994. PAHO was the pioneer in polio eradication in identifying and implementing effective strategies, and in mobilizing Member States and a coalition of donors.

The Global Polio Eradication Initiative is spearheaded by WHO, Rotary International, the US Centers for Disease Control and Prevention and UNICEF (WHO, 2002h). WHO leads the Initiative, with the technical support of the US Centers for Disease Control and Prevention. UNICEF buys vaccines and cold chain equipment. It provides logistical support to ensure that vaccinators can reach all parts of the population. UNICEF staff assists countries with micro-planning for polio eradication activities at the national and district levels. Rotary International has committed more than $510 million to the programme, it has acted as an effective fund-raiser, has mobilized governments and populations and offered volunteers at the operational level.

The Coalition also includes another IGO, the European Commission, – governments of countries affected by polio and donor governments[2] – NGOs (the International Red Cross and Red Crescent movement), other private foundations (the UN Foundation, the Bill and Melinda Gates Foundation), and corporate partners (Aventis Pasteur, De Beers, British Airways). NGOs and volunteers in developing countries play a key role: 10 million volunteers participated in mass immunization campaigns in 2001 alone.

The objectives of the Initiative are:

–　To interrupt transmission of the wild poliovirus as soon as possible and ensure that all WHO regions are certified polio-free or in the process of certification by 2005;[3]
–　To develop polio post-certification policies, including containment of wild poliovirus, global polio-free certification, and the development of a post-certification immunization;
–　To contribute to health systems development by strengthening routine immunization policy and surveillance for communication diseases.

WHO has defined four core strategies to stop transmission of the wild poliovirus and certify all regions polio-free by the end of 2005:

- high infant immunization coverage with four doses of oral polio vaccine in the first year of life;
- supplementary doses of oral polio vaccine to all children under five years of age during national immunization days (NIDs);
- surveillance for wild poliovirus through reporting and laboratory testing of all cases of acute flaccid paralysis among children under fifteen years of age;
- targeted 'mop-up' campaigns once wild poliovirus transmission is limited to a specific focal area.

Before a WHO region can be certified polio-free, four conditions must be certified:

- at least three years of zero polio cases due to wild poliovirus;
- excellent certification standard surveillance;
- each country must illustrate the capacity to detect, report and respond to 'imported' polio cases;
- laboratory stocks must be contained and safe management of the wild virus in Inactivated Polio Vaccine manufacturing sites must be assured before the world can be certified polio-free.

National Immunization Days (NIDs)

The conduct of NIDs involves providing oral polio vaccine to all children under five years of age regardless of immunization status over a period of a few days. For maximum impact, NIDs should be conducted in two rounds, four to six weeks apart during the historic low season of polio transmission, which, in most countries is during the cool, dry season. By flooding all children's intestines simultaneously with vaccine virus and rapidly boosting intestinal and humoral immunity, the wild virus is displaced. When conducted correctly, NIDs interrupt poliovirus circulation in large geographic areas and result in dramatic reductions in polio cases (Birmingham *et al*, 1996).

Surveillance

This refers to monitoring the incidence and transmission of polio at the local, national, regional and global level. Surveillance involves the rapid collection and assessment of stool samples from children who are suspected to have polio. This work begins with reporting suspected polio cases to laboratories by health workers and pediatricians at the local level.

WHO has established a network of 145 laboratories, including 123 national laboratories, supported by 15 regional reference laboratories and seven specialized global laboratories to undertake poliovirus surveillance. The critical function of the network is the accurate and reliable isolation and identification of poliovirus in clinical specimens using standardized techniques and reagents.

Achievements

Overall, since the Global Polio Eradication Initiative was launched, the number of cases has fallen by 99.8 per cent, from an estimated 350,000 cases in 1988 to 483 in 2001 (WHO, 2002h). For the same period, the number of polio-infected countries was reduced from 125 to 10. In 1994, the WHO Region for the Americas (36 countries) was certified polio-free, followed in 2000 by the WHO Western Pacific Region (37 countries and areas including China), and the WHO European Region (51 countries) in June 2002. Widely endemic on five continents in 1988, polio is now found only in parts of Africa and South Asia. Progress from 2000 to 2001 includes a reduction in polio-endemic countries from 20 to 10, and a more than 80 per cent reduction in new cases from 2,979 to 483. Two traditional poliovirus reservoirs, Bangladesh and the Democratic Republic of the Congo found no wild poliovirus in 2001, despite very good surveillance.

WHO and UNICEF have recommended that in all countries with high under-five mortality and where vitamin A deficiency is a public health problem, vitamin A supplements should be provided at the same time as the polio vaccine. In 2001 alone, over 60 countries gave vitamin A during polio national immunization days (NIDs), preventing over 250,000 childhood deaths. A study reported by WHO suggests that, in total, one million childhood deaths have been prevented since 1988 through the provision of vitamin A during NIDs.

Countries at risk

WHO warns that as long as a single child remains infected with poliovirus, children in all countries are at risk of contracting the disease. The poliovirus can easily be imported into a polio-free country and can spread rapidly among non immunized populations. In 2002, 7 countries were known to still have ongoing poliovirus transmission. They are – in order from highest to lowest risk of ongoing transmission beyond 2003 – India, Nigeria, Egypt, Pakistan, Afghanistan, Niger and Somalia.

The spread of the epidemic in northern India in 2002, resulting in a six-fold increase in new cases over 2001, showed that the battle was not over.

Uttar Pradesh was particularly hit, with the state accounting for 64 per cent of all new polio cases worldwide (WHO, 2003a). The epidemic spread from Uttar Pradesh to previously polio-free areas within India and to other countries. The epidemic re-occurred after the number of planned polio vaccination campaigns was reduced in India in 2002. Additionally, as many as 15 per cent of homes were not visited during the vaccination activities which took place in that year. Some resistance to vaccination was also reported by government officials and community leaders: a rumour had spread that the oral vaccine was part of a government population control programme[4] (Waldman, 2003). To stem the epidemic, over 80 million children were to be vaccinated in six Indian states over a six-day period. Over 1.3 million vaccination teams of volunteers and health workers, equipped with nearly 200 million doses of vaccine, went from house to house and worked at booths in communities to reach every child under the age of five. The teams had to cover a country the size of Western Europe in six days. To galvanize communities, Rotary

International and UNICEF worked, in cooperation with the national and Uttar Pradesh governments, with such organizations as Aligarh Muslim University, local leaders, Indian film and cricket stars.

Challenges

Polio eradication faces three main challenges:

- Access: securing access to all children, in spite of geographical obstacles and danger in conflict-affected countries is crucial. In the latter cases, UNICEF has negotiated 'Days of Tranquillity' among warring parties. With the help of the UN Secretary-General and other UN partners, and of the International Red Cross and Red Crescent Movement, UNICEF has obtained special cease-fires to ensure that the polio immunization campaigns could be carried out;
- Funding: Necessary financial resources must be secured to purchase oral polio vaccine (in addition to the financial and in-kind donations), plan and implement national immunization days and mop-up campaigns, and cover surveillance and laboratory costs. According to WHO, the total external financial support needed to the end of 2005 – the new target date for certification – is $1 billion. In November 2002, the funding gap was $275 million. A failure to interrupt transmission in time for certification in 2005 will increase the cost of the programme by an estimated $100 million for every year the programme runs beyond the deadline;
- Political commitment: Sustaining political commitment from the highest levels of government is particularly challenging in the face of a disappearing disease. In polio-endemic countries, personal monitoring by the head of state of the progress towards eradication is key to improving the quality of activities. In polio-free countries, political commitment is needed for sustaining certification standard surveillance and achieving laboratory containment of poliovirus.

Business donations

Two business firms have made donations to the polio campaigns. Aventis Pasteur, the pharmaceutical vaccine manufacturer, has donated 110 million vaccine doses to the Initiative since 1997, targeting its donations to African countries affected by conflicts (WHO, 2002i). In 1999, the diamond mining and trading company De Beers announced its multiyear donation of $2.7 million to help fund National Immunization Days in war-torn Angola. 3.3 million children were to be vaccinated in six rounds of nationwide immunization days (WHO, 1999e). WHO said that there were no strings attached. It would be used for training volunteers and transporting vaccines. The donor, De Beers, has a financial stake in Angola, which produces some 15 per cent of the world's diamonds.

British Airways contributes to the programme through its 'Change for Good' Appeal.[5] In 2002, it donated £7,000 to the polio programme in Zambia.

Donations by Foundations

In 1999, the United Nations Foundation pledged $25 million over seven years to eradicate polio in the Indian sub.continent and Sub-Sahara Africa. The UN Foundation was established by Ted Turner in 1998.[6] It has funded more than 70 UN projects, most in support of projects on women and population, children's health, and the environment. The Bill and Melinda Gates Foundation donated $50 million, also in 1999,channelled through the UN Foundation (WHO, 1999).

However, the major support to the international campaign has been given by Rotary International's PolioPlus programme (Beigbeder, 1997).

Rotary International's PolioPlus

During the 1970s, Rotary International began a search to find a global humanitarian programme in which its members could participate actively, not just by fundraising, but by volunteering in their communities and across the world.[7] Rotary's involvement in polio eradication began in 1979 with a five-year commitment to provide and help deliver polio vaccine to six million children of the Philippines. In the next four years, similar five-year commitments were approved for Haiti, Bolivia, Morocco, Sierra Leone and Cambodia. In 1985, Rotary established its PolioPlus programme, with a pledge of $120 million to fund it. By 2005, Rotary's financial commitment will exceed half a billion dollars. Rotary is the largest non-governmental contributor to the global polio eradication campaign.

Initially, Rotary's role was that of a catalyst, providing money for vaccine and volunteer support to overcome problems associated with distribution. More recently, PolioPlus has funded transportation and other operational costs associated with vaccine delivery, surveillance efforts (including laboratory needs) to identify areas where the virus circulates, and training for healthcare workers and volunteers involved in the immunization process. In 1995, Rotary launched a task force to advocate polio eradication to donor governments, resulting in more than $1.5 billion in polio-specific grants from public sector advocacy. In April 2000, Rotary teamed up with the UN Foundation to carry a financial appeal to the private sector – foundations, corporations, and wealthy individuals – resulting in more than $100 million contributions. Collected funds went to the UN Foundation for distribution to polio eradication projects run by WHO and UNICEF. In February 2002, Rotary announced a Polio Eradication Fundraising Campaign to raise $80 million to contribute to the funding gap, estimated by WHO at $275 million as of April 2002.

Rotary's role is not limited to funding, even though the global campaign is dependent on adequate resources. Rotary is the volunteer arm of the global polio eradication partnership. More than one million Rotarians worldwide have contributed to the programme through local Rotary clubs and districts. Hundreds of thousands of volunteers at the local level are providing support at clinics or mobilizing their communities for immunization. Rotarians have delivered vaccine by camels and helicopters, trucks and motorbikes, staffed immunization posts, raised community awareness of the value of immunization, and helped mobilize 10 million volunteers. Rotary volunteers from polio-endemic countries meet on a regular basis with representatives from their governments and partner agencies to plan and implement polio eradication activities in their countries.

Rotary's donation since 1985, including pledges to 2005, is only second to the first donor, the US through CDC and USAID: the US donation is $598 million, Rotary's is $462 million, and expected to rise to $510 million. Rotary's donation is higher than those of the UK ($341 million), Japan ($200 million), the Netherlands ($110 million) and Germany ($65 million)(UNICEF, 2003).

The Trustees of the Rotary Foundation have affirmed that the global eradication of polio will remain the premier goal of Rotary International and its Foundation 'until the day that the world is certified as being rid of the polio virus'.

Expected benefits of the eradication of polio

From the launch of the global initiative begun in 1988, to the eradication target of 2005, WHO estimates that five million people mainly in the developing world, who would otherwise have been paralyzed, will be walking because they have been immunized against polio (WHO, 2002h). By preventing a debilitating disease, the Initiative gives children and their families a greater chance of leading healthy and productive lives. Following the smallpox eradication precedent, the Initiative has, again, demonstrated that well-planned health interventions can reach even the most remote conflict-affected or poorest areas. Tens of millions of volunteers have been trained to deliver the vaccine and vitamin A, fostering a culture of disease prevention.

The long-term benefits of polio eradication far outweigh the short-term costs. More than $500 million are spent annually on routine polio immunization, whereas approximately $100 million are needed annually over the next years needed to achieve the goal.

The savings of polio eradication are potentially as high as $1.5 billion per year – funds that could be used to address other public health priorities. This amount does not include the immeasurable price paid in human suffering by polio victims and their families. After eradication, no child will be paralyzed or killed by the disease even after immunization stops. Since 1979, the US has been recouping its entire contribution to smallpox eradication every 26 days.

Another major benefit of the Initiative is its reinforcement of primary health care, a paradox for a 'vertical' programme. According to WHO officials (Birmingham *et al*, 1996),

> The strategies and infrastructure developed for this initiative will pave the way for better control of diphtheria, measles, neonatal tetanus and other diseases of public health importance. In addition, disease surveillance in most countries is being strengthened or revitalized as the expertise developed for acute flaccid paralysis surveillance can be applied to other health initiatives.

Furthermore, the global laboratory network set up by WHO to undertake poliovirus surveillance could be used in the future for other important diseases.

Conclusion

The polio eradication campaign is another 'success story', as the onchocerciasis programmes. However, its ambitions and final success are not yet assured: the first goal was to eradicate polio by the year 2000 – this deadline has now been postponed until 2005, mainly because of problems of access to remote areas, rendered more difficult because of local conflicts and refugees' movements but also because of financial or other problems which have reduced the extent of vaccinations and, in some areas, because of resistance to vaccination.

This public-private partnership has, again, joined IGOs, governments, NGOs, business firms and foundations. The donation of vaccine doses by Aventis Pasteur is generous, although it does not equal Merck's commitment to donate Mectizan® 'for as long as necessary, wherever needed, to help bring the onchocerciasis under control as a public health problem'.

Rotary's commitment to retain the eradication of polio as its premier goal 'until the day that the world is certified as being rid of the polio virus' is impressive both in terms of confidence in the eradication programme, and as the assured continuation of PolioPlus' generous and effective contribution to the world-wide campaign.

More generally, the donations of Aventis Pasteur and De Beers, the contributions of the UN Foundation and of the Bill and Melinda Gates Foundation, and the active participation of Rotary International provide welcome additional resources to a programme led by IGOs and mainly financed by governments.

For WHO and UNICEF, the interest of these additional resources is obvious. There is no apparent conflict of interest nor further obligations to Aventis Pasteur on the part of WHO and UNICEF as a result of that pharmaceutical firm's donation of vaccine. Contributions by the US-based foundations Rotary International, UN Foundation and Gates Foundation do not have any direct business link and cannot be the cause of any condemnation of principle. NGOs active in campaigns against 'big pharma' alleged abuses have not targeted the polio programme.

For Aventis Pasteur and de Beers, the benefits of their donations are the promotion of enterprises demonstrating their concern with the fight against a disease affecting public health, and a useful public relations exercise. Another benefit for the pharmaceutical firm Aventis Pasteur is to show its proximity and cooperation with WHO and UNICEF in a humanitarian programme.

For Rotary, the campaign associates this organization of business entrepreneurs to a broad international effort of a humanitarian character. The campaign has a solid technical base, a well-defined strategy, a precise and reachable objective and a well-argued economic rationale, on the lines of the successful smallpox eradication campaign. The illness is of global interest, as the populations in both North and South countries are at risk. Rotary benefits from its cooperation with WHO and UNICEF by the technical approval given to its PolioPlus programme and, more generally by the international legitimacy bestowed by two UN agencies to the US foundation.

In compensation for its contribution, Rotary demands public recognition from the governments concerned. In 1995, the Trustees agreed 'that all PolioPlus grants shall be conditioned on an acceptable plan of government acknowledgement and public recognition to Rotary and no funds shall be released until a specific, detailed plan for government acknowledgement and public recognition of the Rotary Foundation of Rotary International as the donor of the grant is received and determined by the Chairman of the Trustees to be acceptable' (Rotary, 1995).

Well understood self-interest, public relations exercise, philanthropy, tax reduction: whatever the reasons, the additional resources are welcome on the condition that they do not carry any overt or hidden obligation for the organizations in conflict with their public health mandate.

The Global Polio Eradication Initiative is generally recognized as a model of public and private cooperation in pursuit of a humanitarian goal. Can this model be duplicated, and under what conditions?

Notes

1   Rotary is 'an organization of business and professional leaders united worldwide who provide humanitarian service, encourage high ethical standards in all vocations, and help build goodwill and peace in the world'. In more than 160 countries, approximately 1.2 million Rotarians belong to more than 30,000 Rotary clubs.
2   Australia, Austria, Belgium, Canada, Denmark, Finland, Germany, Ireland, Italy, Japan, Luxembourg, Netherlands, Norway, the UK and the USA.
3   The WHO regions are the African region, the region of the Americas, the Eastern Mediterranean region, the European region, the South-East Asian region and the Western Pacific region.
4   Many Indians have feared forced sterilization since it was carried out during the 1975 state of emergency decreed by the government of Prime Minister Indira Gandhi.
5   The 'Change for Good' programme was launched in 1994, collecting foreign currency donated by customers on board British Airways flights. It is run in partnership with UNICEF.
6   On 18 September 1997, R.E. Turner announced his gift of $1 billion in support of UN causes. The UN Secretary-General established the United Nations Fund for International Partnership (UNFIP) in March 1998 to coordinate, channel and monitor contributions from the UN Foundation.
7   Information on PolioPlus is based on data provided by Rotary International's internet site accessed in April 2003.

Chapter 8

Fighting Malaria and Tuberculosis

The global fight against malaria and tuberculosis, as the fight against HIV/AIDS, has enlisted international organizations, governments, NGOs, private sector enterprises and foundations. They have set up or joined public-private partnerships, and have created joint groups for the development of drugs against these diseases. In these initiatives, the private sector has played a necessary and useful role, while debates about the desirable limits of this cooperation with public organizations have again been aired.

Fighting malaria

In October 1998, UNICEF, UNDP, the World Bank and WHO joined forces to launch a new campaign to fight malaria, which kills more than one million people a year. The new programme, called 'Roll Back Malaria', was part of a series of initiatives announced by Dr Gro Harlem Brundtland, who had become Director-General of WHO three months before, in July 1998.

Malaria was not a new concern for WHO. In May 1955, the World Health Assembly had decided that WHO should implement a programme having as its ultimate objective the world-wide eradication of malaria (Beigbeder, 1998:122–131). In 1964, the campaign covered over two-thirds of the world population previously exposed to the disease. However, problems of a technical and operational nature were soon acknowledged: inadequate national health services, particular epidemiological patterns, insecticide resistance or changes in the behaviour of the vector, as well as parasite resistance to drugs, problems of access to certain geographical areas or in war-afflicted countries. In 1967, the World Health Assembly expressed its serious concern and considered it necessary to re-examine the global strategy for malaria eradication. In 1969, the Assembly recognized the failures recorded during the campaign and, in practice, replaced malaria eradication by malaria control. The objective of malaria control is more limited than malaria eradication: it aims at reducing the disease until it is no longer a major public health problem. Control must still be maintained by continuous field work.

In 1994, the UN General Assembly called for preventive action and intensification of the struggle against malaria in developing countries, particularly in Africa (Res. 49/135). In May 1997, WHO and UNESCO agreed to collaborate in assisting countries to implement the Global Malaria Control Strategy.

The impact of malaria

Malaria, together with HIV/AIDS and tuberculosis, is one of the major public health challenges undermining development in the poorest countries in the world. Malaria is a life-theatening parasitic disease transmitted by mosquitos (Roll Back Malaria, 2002).

Approximately 40 per cent of the world's population – mostly those living in the world's poorest countries – is at risk of malaria. The disease was successfully eliminated from most countries with temperate climates during the mid-20th century. Malaria is now found throughout the tropical and sub-tropical regions, and causes more than 300 million acute illnesses, and at least one million deaths annually. Ninety per cent of all deaths due to malaria occur in Africa, south of the Sahara, mostly among young children. Malaria kills an African child every 30 seconds. Pregnant women and their unborn children are particularly vulnerable to malaria, which is a major cause of perinatal mortality, low birth weight and maternal anaemia.

The malaria parasite enters the human host when an infected Anopheles mosquito takes a blood meal inside the person. Malaria symptoms appear 9 to 14 days after the infectious mosquito bite. Typically, malaria produces fever, headache, vomiting and other flu-like symptoms. If drugs are not available for treatment or the parasites are resistant to them, the infection can progress rapidly to become life-threatening.

The Roll Back Malaria campaign (RBM)

In 1997, African leaders, at the annual meeting of the Organization of African Unity, called for action to control malaria. The British government then proposed that malaria feature in discussions among the leaders of the G8 meeting in Birmingham, UK, held from 15–17 May, 1998. The eight leaders supported WHO's initiative to 'Roll Back Malaria', with the aim of halving malaria-associated mortality by 2010 and again by 2015 (Nabarro and Tayler, 1998). In April 2000, heads of State of 44 African countries endorsed RBM's goals in the Abuja Declaration, which also set interim targets and drew up a plan of action for expanding access to to and use of effective interventions. One year later, the first Africa Malaria Day re-affirmed this commitment.

Roll Back Malaria is different from previous efforts to fight malaria by enrolling more partners[1] and broadening the scope of its activities. It works not only through new tools for controlling malaria but also by strengthening the health services of affected populations (WHO, 1998c). The latter argument was to respond to accusations leveled at the WHO malaria eradication campaign to have created a vertical programme, targeted at only one disease, with funds directed to that programme, by-passing the primary health care concept of basic health services. The risk is that the goals of RBM may be over-ambitious, as shown by the following list of set activities:

- strengthening health systems to ensure better delivery of health care, especially at district and community levels;

- ensuring the proper and expanded use of insecticide-treated mosquito nets;
- ensuring adequate access to basic healthcare and training of healthcare workers;
- encouraging the development of simpler and more effective means of administering medicines; such as training of village health workers, mothers and drug peddlers on early and appropriate treatment of malaria, especially for children;
- encouraging the development of more effective and new anti-malaria drugs and vaccines.

RBM's four pillars of action are prompt access to treatment, scaling up the use of insecticide-treated mosquito nets, prevention and control of malaria in pregnant women and emergency response.

Roll Back Malaria will require sustained effort and financing, and strong political commitment over the next decade. An external evaluation carried out in January-March 2002 gave mixed signals (Feachem *et al,* 2002). During Phase I (1998 to mid-2002), there have been major accomplishments in advocacy, resource mobilization and consensus-building around priority interventions. Global spending doubled since 1998. It had been expected that a 'loose' governance structure would avoid the risks inherent in a top-heavy management structure, and increase partners' flexibility to act. However, it had introduced inefficiencies in decision-making and had contributed toward lack of accountability within the partnership. The secretariat, based at WHO headquarters, was seen as more responsive to WHO than to other partners. At the country level, progress had been slow, and few systems were in place to ensure rapid progress in Phase II (mid-2002 to 2007). Countries received inadequate and sometimes inconsistent technical advice. Insufficient attention was given to multi-sectoral approaches to health sector development, especially as regards the role of the private sector. The most urgent message of the Evaluation Team was that the absolute and overriding priority for RBM was to demonstrate a significant reduction in the global burden of malaria by 2007.

The Team recommended the creation of an independent governance board, and that the secretariat should be de-linked from the WHO headquarters Technical Team, and made accountable to that board. There was a feeling among RBM partners that WHO had assumed the leadership of the programme, without giving enough voice to its partners. Altogether, the charge was that RBM had no effective nor accountable governance structure.

The creation of the Global Fund to Fight AIDS, Tuberculosis and Malaria in 2001, as an independent, public-private partnership, raised many hopes of increased support to the combat against those epidemics, including malaria (see 'International financing' in Chapter 5). However, the first awards showed that malaria was treated as the poor relation. In April 2002, $378 million were awarded by the Fund for 40 proposals from 31 countries. About 70 percent went to HIV/AIDS, 20 per cent to tuberculosis, and only 10 per cent to malaria. The total award for malaria in Africa was $22.7 million, or an average of $0.17 per person at risk during the first year of the projects. On the other hand, four countries outside Africa (China, Indonesia, Laos and Sri Lanka), which bear only 3 per cent of the world's malaria burden, would have access to 44 per cent of the malaria funds awarded in the first cycle of funding. It was feared that the current cautionary policy of the Global Fund, which impels it to invest mostly in projects that pursue limited goals, would impede national RBM efforts (Teklehaimanot, Snow, 2002).

Cooperation with pharmaceutical companies

In October 1999, a new alliance was launched between WHO, the Japanese Ministry of Health and Welfare and 12 Japanese pharmaceutical companies (WHO, 1999h). In this public-private venture, molecules in the chemical libraries of the 12 companies were to be tested for anti-malarial activity. Positive results in the test system will be followed up by the UNDP/World Bank/WHO Special Programme for Research and Training in Tropical Diseases (TDR) and any candidate antimalarials discovered would be developed by TDR's virtual drug development operation.

In March 2001, GlaxoSmithKline and WHO signed an agreement for the development of a new treatment for malaria called LAPDAP (WHO, 2001 l). LAPDAP will be made available at a preferential price for public health programmes. Both partners have contributed towards the costs of product development and have set up a joint team to oversee the development of the product. Other supporters of the initiative include the UK Department for International Development and the University of Liverpool. WHO, by means of its TDR Programme, is arranging and providing financial support for clinical trials of LAPDAP. GlaxoSmithKline is responsible for product registrations and manufacture of LAPDAP. The company will commercialize the product in the private sector according to standard local market practice.

In May 2001, WHO and Novartis agreed to provide developing countries with a new treatment for drug resistant malaria (WHO, 2001m). Novartis is providing the new therapy, called Coartem, to WHO for use in developing countries at cost – approximately 10 cents a tablet, amounting to less than $2.50 per full treatment for adults and much less for children. Coartem was added to the WHO Essential Medicines List in April 2002. Coartem is manufactured in China. It was co-developed by Novartis and Chinese researchers at the Institute of Microbiology and Epidemiology in Beijing. Coartem is a combination of a Chinese herb derivative, known as artemether, and lumefantrine.

In areas where multidrug resistant malaria is emerging, Roll Back Malaria advises governments to use Coartem. Researchers found that Coartem was more effective than chloroquine in chloroquine resistant areas, but less effective than some cheaper alternatives (Yamey, 2002). They wondered why Roll Back Malaria did not insist that Novartis conduct proper studies comparing its effectiveness against existing antimalarial regimens, and why was the programme promoting Coartem as a firm line treatment for malaria. The RBM manager replied that Coartem was, at the moment, the best single drug available for treating malaria in countries that have multidrug resistant malaria. Médecins Sans Frontières finds that Coartem, although relatively expensive, has the advantage to being easy to use, as the the combination has been developed as a one-pill co-formulation (MSF, 2002c).

Medicines for Malaria Venture (MMV)

This innovative Venture was established as a Swiss Foundation on 3 November 1999, sited in Geneva (WHO, 1999g). Its creation was facilitated by Roundtable discussions between WHO and pharmaceutical industry leaders organized, since October 1998, at the initiative of the newly appointed Director-General, Dr Gro Harlem Brundtland, showing WHO's new willingness to engage with the private sector. In addition to WHO and the International Federation of Pharmaceutical Manufacturers Association, the main sponsors of the Venture were the governments of the Netherlands, Switzerland and the UK, the World Bank, the Rockefeller Foundation and the Global Forum for Health Research. Support and funding were also provided by the Bill and Melinda Gates Foundation, the Wellcome Trust, and a private sector firm, ExxonMobil Corporation.

The countries most affected by malaria do not have the resources to combat the disease. Vaccines do not exist yet, and medicines are still, at present, the only effective option: they are the major tool in the prevention and cure of malaria. However, with growing resistance to existing drugs, there is urgency to discover new drugs at affordable prices for poor disease endemic countries. The major obstacle to the discovery of new antimalarials is the lack of global investment in drug research and development. The high costs and time needed for R&D, without firm prospects of return upon investment once a drug is fully registered and on the market, are dissuasive to the large pharmaceutical companies.

MMV finds its origin in the failure of the market system to provide the required incentives for wide scale R&D in new medicines to treat malaria. The creation of a public-private partnership aimed at combining the efforts of the pharmaceutical industry, with its knowledge and expertise in drug discovery and development, and the public sector, with its depth of expertise in basic biology, clinical medicine, field experience and its public remit.

The Venture is designed to foster and finance the discovery and development of new, cost-effective and affordable anti-malarial drugs to regulatory approval at a rate of one new registered product every five years, and to facilitate their commercialization (WHO, 2000c). The Venture operates as a non-profit business, independent from WHO, although the Director of the WHO Malaria Control Department is a member of the Board. It is run by a Chief Executive Officer and a Board of up to twelve members, chosen for their scientific, medical and public health expertise in malaria and related fields, their research and management competence as well as their experience in business, finance and fundraising.

The Malaria Vaccine Initiative (MVI)

The Malaria Vaccine Initiative at PATH (Program for Appropriate Technology in Health) was created in 1999 through a $50 million grant from the Bill and Melinda Gates Foundation. PATH is an international non-profit organization dedicated to improving health, especially that of women and children. MVI's mission is to accelerate the development of promising malaria vaccine candidates and ensure their availability and accessibility for the developing world. MVI identifies the most promising vaccines and technologies, and selects and implements partnerships with scientists, vaccinologists, and development projects. MVI works to link government, industry, and academia partners with field trial sites in malaria endemic countries.

MVI has currently nine vaccine development projects worldwide. Some of its partners are GlaxoSmithKline Biologicals, Oxxon Pharmaccines in the UK, Apovia Inc. in Germany and California, the UK Medical Research Council, the US National Institutes for Health, other centers in Gambia, India, Mozambique. MVI works with other vaccine programmes, vaccine development partners and the Global Alliance for Vaccines and Immunization (GAVI), to explore commercialization, procurement, and delivery strategies that will maximize public health sector availability in the countries most affected by malaria (see Chapter 9).

Progress assessment (2003)

According to the *Africa Malaria Report* released in April 2003 by WHO and UNICEF (WHO, 2003b), the death toll from malaria remains outrageously high – with more than 3000 African children dying daily. It also stresses that new effective anti-malarial drugs are not yet accessible to the majority of those who need them and that only a small proportion of children at risk of malaria are protected by highly effective insecticide-treated nets. Carol Bellamy, Executive Director of UNICEF said that malaria kills an African child every 30 seconds, and remains one of the most important threats to the health of pregnant women and their newborns. In part, the Report recommended a greater private sector involvement in the national supply and distribution of quality antimalarial drugs, and insecticide treated nets. The proper use of the nets combined with prompt treatment for malaria at comunity level can reduce malaria transmission by as much as 60 per cent and the overall young child death rate by at least one fifth. Eighteen endemic countries have reduced or eliminated taxes and tariffs on anti-malarial products including mosquito nets and insecticides, helping to make these essential products more accessible.

Fighting tuberculosis

In 1991, the World Health Assembly expressed its concern that three million TB deaths and eight million new cases continued to occur annually. It endorsed a dual approach with a global target of successful treatment of 85 per cent of detected sputum-positive patients and detection of 70 per cent of such cases by the year 2000 (Res. WHA44.8). In 1993, the Assembly declared TB 'a Global Emergency' recognizing that TB remained one of the most important causes of death. The already serious situation was rapidly worsening in both developing and industrialized countries as the result of insufficient priority given to TB programmes, of economic recession, of the appalling conditions in many countries due to war, civil disorders, famine and other calamities, of the spread of HIV infection, and of increased international migration (Res. WHA46.36).

In March 1999, Dr Brundtland launched the *Stop TB* Initiative in partnership with the World Bank, the US Centers for Disease Control and Prevention (CDC), and a coalition of NGOs. The objective of the Initiative is to accelerate TB control by expanding the global coalition of partners beyond the health sector; place TB higher on international political and health agendas; and significantly increase investment in TB control.

In March 2000, the Amsterdam Declaration to Stop TB called for accelerated expansion of control measures and for increased political commitment and financial resources to reach the targets for global TB control by 2005. In May 2000, the World Health Assembly restated this call (Res. WHA53.1). In December 2000, G8 members meeting during the Okinawa Infectious Diseases Conference set the objective of reducing by 50 per cent the rate of tuberculosis prevalence and mortality, to be met by 2010. In May 2003, Médecins Sans Frontières called on G8 leaders meeting in Evian (France) in June, to uphold the commitments they made at previous meetings (MSF, 2003b).

Facts about tuberculosis

TB kills about 2 million people each year (including persons infected with HIV). According to WHO (2002j), more than 8 million people become sick with TB each year. One third of the world's population is currently infected, and 16 million suffer daily from active TB. 95 per cent of TB cases and 98 per cent of TB deaths occur in developing countries. Every year, over 1.5 million people acquire active in sub-Saharan Africa. TB spreads through the air and is highly contagious. On average, a person with infectious TB infects 10–15 others every year. People infected with TB do not necessarily become ill – the immune system creates a barrier around the bacilli which can remain dormant for years. Ten per cent of infected people (who do not have HIV/AIDS) develop active TB at some point during their lifetime. Patients develop a persistent cough (sometimes with blood in the sputum), fever, weight loss, chest pain and breathlessness.

The spread of TB is linked in part with the more frequent travel of people, and forced migration. HIV is accelerating the spread of TB: TB is a leading cause of death among people with HIV/AIDS. In Africa, three quarters of TB patients are HIV-infected. TB affects refugees and displaced persons in crowded camps and shelters.

WHO strategy

In 1993, WHO set global goals of detecting 70 per cent of all infectious TB cases and treating 85 per cent of those cases with the WHO recommended treatment for the year 2000. This target was not reached, and WHO urged a concerted effort to meet the target by 2005. The WHO recommended treatment strategy for detection and cure of TB is DOTS. DOTS combines five elements: political commitment, case detection through sputum smear microscopy, directly observed short-term treatment, regular drug supplies and monitoring systems. Once infectious cases have been detected using microscopy services, health and community workers and trained volunteers observe and record patients swallowing the correct dosage of anti-TB medicines, and document that the patient has been cured.

The most common anti-TB drugs are isoniazid, rifampicin, pyrazinamide, streptomycin and ethambutol. Treatment lasts from six to eight months. Sputum smear testing is repeated after two months, to check progress, and again at the end of the treatment.

Since DOTS was introduced on a global scale in 1991, about 10 million patients have received treatment. DOTS produces cure rates of up to 95 per cent, even in the poorest countries. It prevents new infections by curing infectious patients. DOTS prevents the development of multidrug-resistant TB (MDR-TB) by ensuring the full course of the treatment. A six-month supply of drugs for DOTS costs approximately $10 per patient in some countries. Drug-resistant TB is caused by inconsistent or partial treatment by patients who do not take their drugs regularly for the required period because they start to feel better. It may also be caused by the prescription of the wrong treatment regimens, or by an unreliable drug supply. TB bacilli may be resistant to specific drugs. The most dangerous form of drug-resistant TB is multidrug-resistant TB, which is defined as due to TB bacilli resistant to at least isoniazid and refampicin, the two most powerful anti-TB drugs. Rates of MDR-TB are high in some countries, especially in the former Soviet Union, and threaten control efforts. Drug-resistance is treatable, but may require extensive and expensive chemotherapy.

The Global Alliance for TB Drug Development

The Alliance, created in 2000, is a not-for-profit public-private partnership aimed at accelerating the discovery and development of faster-acting and affordable drugs to fight TB. Its partners find that the global health community is not equipped to confront the current triple threat: exponential rapid spread of TB infection, rise of drug-resistant strains and interaction with the HIV/AIDS epidemic. Faster-acting drugs would provide simpler therapeutic and prophylactic regimens. The Alliance is building up a portfolio of promising drug candidates by forging innovative partnerships for their development. It expects to register an effective new drug by 2010 that will shorten the duration of TB treatment, or simplify its completion, be effective against MDR-TB and improve the treatment of latent TB infection. The Alliance is governed by a Board of Directors of seven to thirteen members, representing international and national government agencies, pharmaceutical and biotechnology companies, private foundations and NGOs. Its membership currently includes one WHO official, and representatives from Eli Lilly, Chiron and the Rockefeller Foundation.

By 2002, the Alliance had raised $40 million from the Rockefeller Foundation and the Bill and Melinda Gates Foundation (McManus and Saywell, 2002). With funds, it buys the worldwide rights to promising drugs and outsources research and development to public laboratories or industry.

In February 2002, it licensed a potential new drug candidate called PA-824 from Chiron Corporation, the US-based company (Palmedo, 2002). Companies like Chiron are given the option to license back their drugs to sell in wealthier countries. If they exercise the option, they have to repay the Alliance all fees and R&D investments, plus royalties. The Alliance retains all rights to the rest of the world and Chiron receives no royalties for any products in these countries.

The agreement between the Alliance and Chiron was the first such arrangement between a private sector company and a non-profit organization for a new compound that could treat TB. According to the terms of the Memorandum of Understanding, the Alliance will undertake further development of PA-824, which was in preclinical development, and a family of nitroimidazoles derivatives. The Alliance will undertake further development of PA-824, and /or of its analogs licensed from Chiron. In addition, provisions have been made for possible further collaboration with Chiron at later stages of development, including a grant-back option to Chiron for manufacture and commercialization of products in developed markets. The parties have agreed that no royalties will be due under the agreement for drugs marketed in less developed economies, including impoverished countries with a high burden of TB.

Other contributions by pharmaceutical companies

In 2000, Eli Lilly announced a deal with WHO to supply high-priced antibiotics to combat drug-resistant TB in Russia and other countries. Its drugs would be used in a pilot project to treat and monitor about 1,000 Russian prisoners and some civilians infected with TB resistant to conventional drug treatments. The project might be expanded to other parts of Russia, as well as Latvia, Estonia, Peru, the Philippines, Morocco, Chile and other regions where multi-drug-resistant TB is becoming a public health crisis. Eli Lilly would provide some quantity of capromycin and cycloserine at reduced prices.

In 2001, public health experts and scientists from WHO, Harvard Medical School, Médecins Sans Frontières (MSF) and other partners worked together to reduce the prices for MDR-TB drugs by 48–97 percent, by defining the market, negotiating bulk purchases with suppliers, and ensuring rational use of the drugs (WHO *Bulletin,* 2001). Acting as a negotiator for the parties, MSF consolidated the various sources of demand, negotiated prices, provided advance funds for bulk purchase and assisted with technical support. WHO created a regulatory mechanism called the 'Green Light Committee' to promote access to the drugs.

As a result, Eli Lilly will sell capreomycin, which normally costs up to $25 per dose, to MSF for as little as $1, a 96 percent discount. The price of cycloserine went down by 96 per cent from $3.38 to $0.14. The drug was only available from one supplier. The cost of ofloxacin, because of competition through tendering went down by 87.25 per cent from $2.60 to $0.33. Jacobuy Pharmaceuticals, a small US company, will offer a 40 percent discount on para-amino-salicylic acid. Under the new agreement, the overall price from treating an MDR-TB patient will amount to less than $3,000, instead of $15,000.

In February 2003, Novartis said that it was establishing a research center in Singapore, with support from the Singapore government, the Novartis Institute for Tropical Diseases (Normile, 2003). It involves an investment of $122 million. The Institute, a private, non-profit institution, will initially focus on multidrug-resistant TB and dengue. Any resulting drugs will be available to developing countries without royalties. At the same time, the Institute will give Novartis an entry into the medical and regulatory environments of developing countries.

As another contribution, Novartis will donate 100,000 DOTS treatments to TB every year for a five year period starting in 2003, as a contribution to the Global Fund to Fight HIV/AIDS, TB and Malaria. The donation will be provided to selected African countries where it can make a significant contribution to improve the TB situation in the country.

In June 2001, the British-Swedish pharmaceutical firm AstraZeneca announced plans to set up a research center focusing on new treatments for TB in Bangalore (India). Britain's GlaxoSmithKline is also working on the disease.

Progress assessment (2003)

In March 2003, WHO announced that over 10 million TB patients had been successfully treated under DOTS (WHO, 2003c). The growth of TB incidence rate had slowed to 0.4 per cent per year. The number of countries that have adopted the TB control strategy had grown to 155 countries – of 192 WHO Member States –, and more than 60 per cent of the world's population now had access to DOTS services.

However, the WHO report found that the TB epidemic was still growing unabated in sub-Saharan countries, where TB is closely linked with HIV/AIDS and poverty,and in many of the Newly Independent States born of the break-up of the former Soviet Union, where it is exacerbated by poverty and social disruption. In some high-HIV countries of sub-Saharan Africa, TB rates have quadrupled since the 1980s and threaten to overwhelm well-established control programmes.

Conclusion

Since 1998, WHO, UNICEF and other partners have launched well-publicized campaigns against well-known enemies of public health, malaria and TB. These new campaigns, Roll Back Malaria and Stop TB gave new life and impetus to past efforts, and gave more visibility to forgotten diseases hitting mainly the populations of developing countries (malaria), or North and South countries, in view of a link to HIV/AIDS (tuberculosis). Both campaigns have a similar objective, disease control, forgetting the over-ambitious and unrealistic objective of eradication.

The methods are similar to those already applied for HIV/AIDS: identify the enemy, the causes of its spread, apply existing measures more systematically: for malaria, a more effective treatment (Coartem), more use of insecticide-treated bednets, – for TB, better detection, use of DOTS. At the same time, encourage laboratories to initiate or develop research on vaccine and drugs, apply pressure on pharmaceutical companies to reduce their prices for developing countries.

In all cases, the campaigns are based on broad alliances with different memberships, but generally including the international organizations (WHO and UNICEF), the World Bank, willing governments, NGOs (MSF, Oxfam), foundations (The UN Foundation, the Gates Foundation, the Soros Open Society Institute, the Rockefeller Foundation), and private sector enterprises.

Medicines for Malaria Venture deviated from these now classical alliances by setting up a national (Swiss) foundation, as a non-profit organization independent from its creators, WHO, the World Bank, IFPMA and others. A national foundation with international objectives and scope, MMV, in its own sphere, has characteristics similar to those of the International Committee of the Red Cross in the humanitarian field. MMV's independence and competence gives it the flexibility needed to promote the discovery and development of new, cost-effective and affordable anti-malarial drugs, a long-neglected area.

Cooperation of international organizations, and preferably not conflict, with the private sector is essential for research and development of new vaccines and more effective drugs, and to obtain preferential prices for public health programmes. However, the pharmaceutical industry's belated willingness to reduce prices was not due to a conversion of profit-making companies to a philanthropic stance: it was a result of wide and strong public pressures by NGOs which caused the retreat of the industry in South Africa in 2001: bad publicity may affect profits. The pharmaceutical industry has started to realize that their commercial interests go beyond the short-term satisfaction of their shareholders and obtaining quick profits. Shareholders and the general public also include present or future patients, and have started applying pressure on the companies to honour their self-proclaimed 'social responsibility'. Their own self-interest is also to work with, and not against, the international organizations concerned with public health, which give legitimacy to their common programmes.

The international organizations benefit from the alliances by extending the scope of their programmes, obtaining additional resources, benefiting from NGOs pressures on price reduction and access to medicines. WHO also plays a role in establishing standards, defining strategies and acting as a facilitator between NGOs and the industry, while trying to maintain some distance from them. It should not show any preference for the products of any company, except on strictly technical, well-established grounds. WHO should ensure that ethical conditions are applied to new drug testing.

Foundations help by offering donations or funding for specific projects, by supporting specific public health programmes. While often created by business leaders or firms, they have no direct link with any specific commercial enterprise and do not promote their interests. Their contributions to both the malaria and TB programmes are appreciated.

NGOs play their usual 'activist' role in publicizing the need for action mainly in developing countries, prodding rich countries to pay more and international organizations to be more assertive publicly in their promotion of 'health for all' and access to medicines.

Note

1   Besides UNICEF, UNDP, the World Bank and WHO, partners include the European Union, the African Development Bank, USAID, the US Centers for Disease Control and Prevention (CDC), the Canadian International Development Agency, the UK Department for International Development, The UN Foundation, the NGO Médecins Sans Frontières and Exxon Mobil Corporation.

Chapter 9

Vaccines and Immunization

The Global Alliance for Vaccines and Immunization (GAVI) was created in 1999 in response to stagnating immunization rates and widening global disparities in access to vaccines. It focuses on increasing access to vaccines among children in poor countries. Vaccines are the most cost effective public health interventions but there are wide variations in essential vaccine coverage between North and South countries and within regions. Children in the developed countries have access to newer, more effective and more expensive vaccines to protect them against major childhood diseases. But in sub-Saharan Africa only half of the children have access to basic immunization against common diseases such as tuberculosis, measles, tetanus and whooping cough. In poor and isolated areas of developing countries, vaccines reach fewer than one in twenty children (WHO, 2002k).

GAVI is another public-private partnership for health, whose partners include governments, UNICEF, WHO, the World Bank, the Bill and Melinda Gates Foundation, the vaccine industry, public health institutions and NGOs. For the first time, business agents (vaccine manufacturers in this case) are full partners in these schemes, with representatives on the GAVI Board, the Board of the Vaccine Fund and implementing groups. Another specificity is that it has adopted a business-approach to funding health programmes in developing countries.

GAVI is not the first partnership in this field. It is the outcome of many international public health initiatives and the successor of the Children's Vaccine Initiative (CVI). It was preceded and followed by other vaccine initiatives related to specific diseases: poliomyelitis, HIV/AIDS, malaria and measles.

Previous international efforts

In the 1960s, there was no systematic notification of vaccination coverage rates or vaccine quality, in particular in developing countries, and, finally, vaccination programmes were rarely included in the activities of national health services.

In 1974, the World Health Assembly created the Expanded Programme on Immunization (EPI) and recommended that WHO Member States develop or maintain immunization and surveillance programmes against some or all of the following diseases: diphtheria, pertussis, tetanus, measles, poliomyelitis, tuberculosis, smallpox, and others, where applicable, according to the epidemiological situation in their respective countries.

In September 1978, the International Conference convened jointly by UNICEF and WHO adopted the Alma-Ata Declaration. The Declaration included immunization against the major infectious diseases as one of the eight elements required, so that, by the year 2000, all mankind could benefit from primary health care.

In 1974, coverage for children under one year of age in developing countries was well below five per cent. In 1987, for the first time in history, coverage exceeded 50 per cent for all vaccines except measles (at 46 per cent). By 1991, WHO and UNICEF reported that the goal of immunizing 80 per cent of the world's children had been achieved. This had resulted in more than three million deaths from the EPI diseases being averted each year.

In a WHO report issued in 1994, the Global Advisory Group[1] concluded that the success of the global EPI represented 'one of the most important public health triumphs of this century and [was] a major contribution towards the global target of Health for All'. The Group was however concerned by the failure to move beyond the 80 per cent coverage target achieved in 1990 and the reductions in coverage in some countries on every continent. The problem of 'reaching the unreached' was particularly important in Africa. The World Development Report 1993 'Investing in Health' issued by the World Bank had identified immunization as one of the most cost-effective public health interventions (Beigbeder, 2001:79–80).

The Children's Vaccine Initiative (CVI)

The Children's Vaccine Initiative (CVI) was launched at the World Summit for Children in New York in 1990 by four international organizations, UNICEF, UNDP, WHO and the World Bank, and the Rockefeller Foundation. It involved governments, NGOs, industry and research groups. Its motivation was that the global progress of children's immunization was hampered by various problems with the existing vaccines: the vaccines were not totally effective, they were often given too late to be potent, they often lacked the ability to tolerate tropical heat and they required multiple shots that necessitated complex delivery systems.

The Declaration of New York, signed by the participants of the World Summit for Children on 10 September 1990, called on the world to use current science to make new and better vaccines. The vaccines should be given in one or two doses, given early in life, combined in unusual ways so as to reduce the number of injections, to be more heat stable, to be useful against a wide variety of diseases and to be affordable. In addition, investments should be made to simplify production and quality control methods, support field trials, speed licensing and help production in developing countries. The Declaration called on world leaders to 'commit themselves to a children's vaccine initiative that aims to produce and deliver "ideal" children's vaccines'.

In 1991, it was decided that CVI would take the form of an independent entity sited in Geneva, but not led by WHO.

CVI was not a new institution, but a network and a global think tank for vaccines and immunization. It aimed at improving the global supply and quality of existing vaccines, facilitating a dialogue between the public and private sectors on the research and development of new vaccines, and developing strategies to ensure that these vaccines will be affordable for use in developing countries. CVI was to build a global forum to include development agencies, governments, donors, public sector and commercial vaccine manufacturers, vaccine researchers and national immunization programme managers. The intent was that, through establishing a dialogue between all key players in the global vaccine system – from research, testing, licensing and production to quality control, vaccine procurement and delivery – CVI would be able to identify weaknesses and potential bottlenecks in the system and seek workable solutions.

Under the CVI-run Vaccine Independence Initiative, countries were required to rigorously plan for their vaccine needs and vaccine budget over a two- and five-year period. The Initiative was to assist developing countries to procure vaccines through the UNICEF system and to pay for the vaccines either in local or hard currencies. The establishment in 1994 of the Global Programme for Vaccines and Immunization (GPV) at the WHO headquarters reflected the new priorities identified by CVI. The new programme integrated two operational units: EPI and the Vaccine and Development Unit and created a third, the Vaccine Supply and Quality Unit. CVI was instrumental in the creation of the International Vaccine Institute in Seoul, Korea, uniquely dedicated to research, development and capacity-building in the field of vaccines.

The decision to disband CVI and replace it by GAVI was taken during a meeting in Bellagio, in March 1999, where dissensions appeared between WHO, the World Bank and other partners. In April 1999, the Chief Executive Officers of Pasteur Mérieux Connaught, Merck Vaccines, Wyeth Vaccines and SmithKline Beecham Biologicals wrote to WHO, the World Bank and UNICEF to express their disappointment as to the failure of discussions held in the previous twelve months with a view to finding ways to improve children's immunization in the poorest countries.

The Children's Vaccine Program (CVP)

In 1998, the Program for Appropriate Technology in Health (PATH) launched this Program with a commitment by the Bill & Melinda Gates Foundation of $100 million. Building on the WHO EPI programme, its mission is to promote equal access to new vaccines worldwide. and to introduce new vaccines and immunization technologies. Its partners are the World Bank, WHO, UNICEF, UNDP, the Children's Vaccine Initiative, the International Vaccine Institute.

Vaccine initiatives related to specific diseases

The Global Initiative to eradicate poliomyelitis was launched by the World Health Assembly in 1988 (see Chapter 7). The programme is based on increasing the immunization coverage of children under five years of age with the effective oral polio vaccine.

The International AIDS Vaccine Initiative (IAVI) was created in 1996 by Dr. Seth Berkley, an organization working to speed the research, development and distribution of preventive AIDS vaccines (see 'Vaccine initiatives' in Chapter 5). Its partners are the World Bank, policy leaders and industry leaders, governments, scientists and foundations. It has created the AIDS Vaccine Development Partnership. It has laid the foundation for national AIDS vaccine programmes and is associated with vaccine tests in several countries.

Left aside by IAVI, WHO and UNAIDS created in February 2000 their HIV Vaccine Initiative to promote the development of an AIDS vaccine. It has elaborated the framework to conduct vaccine tests under strict ethical and scientific standards.

The Malaria Vaccine Initiative at PATH (MVI) was created in 1999 through another grant from the Gates Foundation, in an amount of $50 million (see 'The Malaria Vaccine Initiative' in Chapter 8). It has currently nine vaccine development projects worldwide. It works with other vaccine programmes, vaccine development partners and GAVI. It aims at linking government, industry and academia partners with field trial sites in malaria endemic countries.

The Measles Initiative is a US-based partnership which includes the American Red Cross, the United Nations Foundation, the US Centers for Disease Control and Prevention, UNICEF, WHO and the Pan American Health Organization. African partners include national Ministries of Health, national Red Cross and Red Crescent Societies with the support of the International Federation of Red Cross and Red Crescent Associations, and other NGOs. Created in February 2002 at the initiative of the American Red Cross, the Initiative is a long-term commitment to control measles deaths, beginning in Africa, by supporting immunization programmes, including vaccinating 200 million children through both mass and follow-up campaigns in up to 36 Sub-Saharan African countries, preventing 1.2 million deaths over five years (UNICEF, 2002a).

The Global Alliance for Vaccines and Immunization (GAVI)

The Alliance was created in 1999 to coordinate a global network of international development organizations, governments, multilateral development banks, philanthropic organizations, private sector leaders and others in re-energizing the global commitment to vaccines and immunization. GAVI sees immunization as a fundamental cornerstone of global health, a key component of economic development, and an essential first step in enabling each child to reach his or her fullest physical and intellectual potential (WHO, 2000d).

The official justification for the creation of GAVI was based on a one-year review of immunization-related activities undertaken by the major interested parties of CVI, which identified the following major gaps:

– stagnant immunization programmes with a decline in the basic EPI coverage for certain diseases as well as marked regional discrepancies;
– delay in the introduction of newly developed, highly efficacious vaccines against major killers such as Hepatitis B, haemophilus influenza b and yellow fever into the poorest countries;
– limited investment into vaccine research for diseases with high burden in developing countries in preference to diseases in developed countries with lesser global importance but higher financial value (Beigbeder, 2001:83–86).

The Alliance has set five strategic objectives:

– Improving access to sustainable immunization services;

- Expanding the use of all existing safe and cost-effective vaccines;
- Accelerating the development and introduction of new vaccines;
- Accelerating research and development efforts on vaccines and related products specifically needed by developing countries, especially those against HIV/AIDS, malaria and tuberculosis;
- Making immunization coverage an integral part of the design and assessment of international development efforts, including deep debt relief.

As noted above, GAVI is the first international public-private partnership in which private sector agents, in this case vaccine manufacturers, are full partners, with representatives on the GAVI Board and implementing groups. The Board sets the policies of the Alliance. It has five renewable members – WHO, UNICEF, the World Bank, The Vaccine Fund and the Bill & Melinda Gates Foundation. The current President of the The Vaccine Fund, Jacques-François Martin, was a former CEO of Parteurop, a biotech consulting company, of Rhone-Poulenc Pharma in Hamburg and of Pasteur-Mérieux. The Board has twelve additional, rotating members.[2] Among the latter, three were also business-related members in 2003: the Executive Vice-President of Wyeth Pharmaceuticals, the Director-General of the Serum Institute of India, as a developing country vaccine industry, the Director-General of the Institut Pasteur, as a research institute.

Reflecting the UN's and WHO's opening to the private sector, GAVI launched its vaccination campaign, 'The Children's Challenge', on 31 January 2000 at the World Economic Forum in Davos, the meeting place of business and political leaders. GAVI partners outlined three main inequities that need to be addressed in order to achieve the goal of universal immunization:

- the 30 million children born every year in poor countries who are still not receiving the 'basic six' immunizations;
- the growing disparity in the number of vaccines available to children in industrialized and developing countries;
- the lack of investment in poorer countries, particularly HIV/AIDS, malaria and tuberculosis.

At the Davos meeting, business leaders from the vaccine/pharmaceutical industry promised to accelerate the delivery of available but under-utilized vaccines for yellow fever, hepatitis B and Hib. Jean-Jacques Bertrand, a member of the GAVI Board said: 'As global corporations, employers, and suppliers of vaccine, the pharmaceutical industry as represented by the International Federation of Pharmaceutical Manufacturers Associations (IFPMA) has taken a far-sighted role in support of the Children's Challenge ... Individual companies that are participating in the GAVI efforts have pledged to continue to provide vaccines of the highest quality and to actively develop new breakthrough vaccines'.

IFPMA has declared that its vaccine industry members[3] will, in cooperation with their GAVI partners, work to ensure accessibility to vaccines for all the world's children with particular focus on the poorest people and countries (GAVI, 2002a). On behalf of the five vaccine manufacturers that he represented on the GAVI Board in the period 2000–2002, Bertrand announced that the global vaccine industry would support GAVI in five key areas:

- the supply of high quality vaccines to the world's poorest populations;
- investment in the development and supply of new breakthrough vaccines on a worldwide basis;
- development of technologies to facilitate the distribution and administration of vaccines within countries;
- contribute to the education of immunization providers in those countries; and,
- engage other private sector organizations in the mission of GAVI.

Aventis Pasteur went further: it said that it was committed to its legacy of public health and would continue to supply developing countries with vaccines at tiered prices, under specific conditions, to help improve access to vaccines and reduce the present lag time between introduction of new vaccines in industrialized and developing countries. 'Tiered-pricing' is a strategy that sets vaccine prices at different levels for different markets according to levels of income. Aventis Pasteur has long been one of UNICEF's largest vaccine suppliers. It has sponsored the distribution of GAVI's Immunization Resource kit. This collection of documents, video clips, and computer presentations is aimed at providing countries with advocacy, and related resources, for improving immunization programmes (Aventis (undated)).

The Global Fund for Children's Vaccines

In November 1999, the Bill & Melinda Gates Foundation donated $750 million over five years to establish the Global Fund for Children's Vaccines. The Fund is a financing mechanism designed to help the Alliance achieve its objectives by raising new resources and channeling them to developing countries. With low administrative costs, approximately 98 per cent of the Fund's resources go directly to countries. The Fund's total resources were, in 2003, above $1 billion for 2001–2005. In addition to the Gates Foundation's donation, commitments have been received from the governments of Norway, the UK, the USA, the Netherlands, Denmark and Sweden, and from the private sector.

Governments in the 74 poorest countries (GNP below $1000 per capita) are eligible to apply for support. By the end of 2002, 66 of these countries had applied and 54 countries had been approved. The Vaccine Fund and GAVI have made five-year commitments of more than $800 million to these countries. Of that, approximately two-thirds is used to purchase vaccines and supplies and the rest is for support for capacity development and public health infrastructure.

An additional purpose of the Fund is to demonstrate to vaccine manufacturers that a developing country market exists for newer vaccines. GAVI partners are hoping that this will encourage manufacturers to increase current vaccine production, and develop new and even better vaccines in the future.

The Board of Directors of the Vaccine Fund has currently 14 members.[4] Business is represented by the President of the Vaccine Fund, Jacques-François Martin, and by George W. Wellde, from the Goldman Sachs Group.

A business-like approach

No doubt under the influence of its business-related partners and of the Gates Foundation, GAVI introduced a new idea in international development: outcome-based grants that give governments responsibility and autonomy to decide how money is used: if they do not show results, the funding stops (UNICEF, 2002b). GAVI wants recipient countries to take the initiative and manage their own program. GAVI pays for the vaccines, then monitors progress. It cuts funds for countries that do not do enough to meet targets. To ensure accountability, an initial effort to audit country data was undertaken in 2001 by an independent consortium that included the international auditing firm, Deloitte Touche Tomatsu.

While traditional health initiatives often start off by hand-picking countries to participate in a pilot project – a slow process – GAVI lets any country apply, as long as it is one of the 74 poorest countries. In 2002, 66, or 90 per cent of eligible countries, had applied for Vaccine Fund support and the applications of 53 countries had been approved, including some in the most difficult situations such as Sierra Leone, Liberia and Afghanistan.

Achievements

Since its launch in Davos in January 2000, according to UNICEF, one of the major achievements of GAVI and the Vaccine Fund is a new vaccine procurement system. By guaranteeing long-term purchasing commitments, it enables manufacturers to produce vaccines at affordable prices. In this way, a viable market has been created combining new and old antigens, such as hepatitis B combined with DTP. However, it was found in 2002 that demand for the new combination vaccines vastly oustripped supply: monovalent vaccines were shipped instead. It was also found that a situation of monopoly existed: only one manufacturer, GlaxoSmithKline, was able to fill orders for combination vaccines. It was however predicted that in the coming years several other manufacturers would produce and offer these vaccines. 'Stronger country forecasts and stable funding are the pillars for securing vaccines from industry', said Carol Bellamy, GAVI Board Chair and Executive Director of UNICEF (GAVI, 2002b). UNICEF manages the procurement and delivery of vaccines for GAVI.

In April 2001, GAVI began the first round of a global schedule of vaccine delivery to Mozambique, the first to reach the African continent (UNICEF, 2001). The Mozambican government received the first half of 1.3 million doses of DTP-hepB vaccines worth an estimated $1.5 million. An additional contribution of $462,000 to strengthen immunization services was also awarded. The Boane District in the country would pilot immunization with the combination DTP-hepB vaccines until a nation-wide campaign began in July 2001. The pilot was to set in motion a host of immunization activities including: training health workers about the new combination vaccine and correct use of safety devices, and how to communicate with a variety of audiences the importance of all infants receiving a full schedule of vaccinations.

In addition to the vaccines themselves, auto-disposable syringes and safety boxes were also provided. This syringe includes a safety device that prevents its re-use.

WHO, UNICEF, UNFPA and the Federation of Red Cross and Red Crescent Associations have adopted a global policy on injection safety calling for the use of those syringes for all immunization by the end of 2002.

In 2001, Mozambique was one of 25 countries to secure support from GAVI and the Global Fund. Mozambique has one of the highest rates of child mortality in the world with 146 out of 1,000 children dying before their first birthday.

In June 2002, the GAVI Board noted that 60 out of the 75 eligible countries were now supported by the Alliance. The Vaccine Fund had already committed nearly $1 billion in immunization programmes financing over five years.

By November 2002, 130 million vaccine doses had been delivered to countries. According to preliminary estimates by WHO, the vaccines provided by GAVI and the Vaccine Fund had already saved more than 100,000 lives.

A report released in November 2002, 'The State of the World's Vaccines and Immunization Report', still warned that if urgent and strategic action was not taken to close the gaps in funding, research and global immunization coverage, the world would see the re-introduction of old diseases and the emergence of new infections (WHO, 2002 l). Low donor investment was one of the major reasons for the huge gaps in coverage. Another factor cited for the low vaccination coverage was the low level of investment in immunization by developing countries. The report underscored the urgent need for vaccines against malaria, and a new vaccine for tuberculosis.

In February 2003, GAVI and the Vaccine Fund announced that Johns Hopkins Bloomberg School of Public Health and the Program for Appropriate Technology in Health (PATH) had been selected to each receive a $30 million grant to ensure that vaccines against pneumococcus and rotavirus were made available to developing countries quickly once they were licensed (GAVI, 2003). It is estimated that every year half a million children die as a result of rotavirus-related diarrhoea, and one million from pneumococcus-related pneumonia. Both grants would be used to bring together experts in research, regulation, marketing and manufacturing to address potential obstacles such as lack of disease burden data and vaccine efficacy, uncertain market demand, and regulatory processes that could delay approval of vaccines for the developing world.

Critical assessments

The operations of GAVI and of the Vaccine Fund were reviewed at the first biannual meeting of GAVI partners held in Noordwijk (The Netherlands) from 20–21 November 2000. An analysis by Dr Anita Hardon, head of the Medical Anthropology Unit at the University of Amsterdam, found that 'the emphasis on the introduction of new and under-used vaccines in GAVI reflected a more general shift away from equity towards technological innovation and disease eradication in global health programmes' (Hardon, 2001). In her view, 'Now in the opening days of the new millenium, international health policy makers involved in immunization programmes seem to view developing countries no longer primarily as recipients of internationally procured essential vaccines, but rather, as markets for new ones'. She recalled the conditions set for industry participation in the Alliance by Jean Stephenne, President of SmithKline Biologicals (a company producing the DTP-hepatitis combination now in great demand), outlined in one of the meeting's keynote speeches. This included a guarantee for 'reasonable prices', support for a credible and sustainable market, respect for international property rights, a tiered pricing system including safeguards against re-export of products back from developing countries to high-priced markets, and a prohibition on compulsory licensing. In plenary sessions, industry representatives said that they opposed technology transfer proposals. Hardon noted that in GAVI, UN agencies are partners and no longer the leaders. Decisions are made in the Board which is dominated by donors and Northern representatives. GAVI's structure includes no clear mechanisms for accountability nor is there transparency in its decision-making. She expressed concern about the lack of sustainability: under GAVI, donor dependence for the procurement of vaccines is being reinforced.

In an interview with the BMJ (Yamey, 2001), Hardon said that the inclusion of pharmaceutical industry in the Alliance creates a possible conflict of interest, as the industry's interest in marketing new products could be at odds with the overall aims of the Alliance.

According to a representative from the Malaria Vaccine Initiative, pharmaceutical companies want to get paid in the range of $10 per dose of vaccine, while UNICEF and WHO want prices counted in pennies so that poor countries can afford these vaccines (Paulson, 2001). Business partners on the GAVI Board may leave if the Alliance supported the creation of competitors in developing countries.

Responding to some of these concerns, Dr Tore Godal, Executive Secretary of GAVI, said: 'The goal is that by 2005, 80 per cent of districts in 80 per cent of countries will have full vaccination coverage. This addresses the question of equity'. GAVI increased the proportion of its annual budget allocated to immunization systems to 30 per cent from a first year level of 10 per cent. Godal believed that, even though the Alliance involves industry, conflicts of interest are avoided because UNICEF is responsible for procuring vaccines via a 'competitive, open process of bidding'. The Alliance is accountable to the boards of UN agencies, and it has an independent technical review committee made up largely of public health experts in the developing world.

Other questions or criticisms of GAVI concerned the scope and technical aspects of the Alliance, rather than the role of business enterprises in this type of partnership.

For instance, the Children's Vaccine Program and the Malaria Vaccine Initiative are financed by Gates and are part of GAVI (Paulson, 2001). The International AIDS Vaccine Initiative is partially funded by Gates but is not part of GAVI. WHO's polio eradication campaign is not part of GAVI although its aims overlap with those of the Alliance. How should all these programmes work together, avoiding duplication and destructive competition? Should GAVI stay focused mostly on childhood diseases or join the existing vaccine efforts on AIDS, malaria and tuberculosis? Should GAVI support disease eradication efforts, such as the polio and measles campaigns, or is it better to emphasize re-building failing public health and immunization systems? What is the best way to measure success in disease control efforts?

A study published by the London School of Hygiene and Tropical Medicine and Save the Children UK in 2002 reviewed and reported on the country level experience of GAVI in four countries (Brugha, Starling, Walt, 2002). It found that countries welcomed the introduction of hepatitis B vaccine, safe injection equipment, and the financial support to strengthen immunization programmes. All reported that the pace of the application process was too rapid. District visits revealed low staffing levels, insufficient transport and fuel, poorly functioning cold chains, and infrequent supervision. Information systems were unreliable, which would be an obstacle to GAVI when monitoring and rewarding improvements in immunization coverage. Also, the high cost of expensive new vaccines will be difficult to sustain if GAVI funding stops at the end of the five-year commitment.

Based on this study, an analysis paper by Save the Children UK, published in January-March 2002, raised several concerns about GAVI's mode of operation (Save the Children UK, 2002). Although not investigated by the study, the role of business partners in the Alliance was identified as an issue of concern:

> ... on its Board sit parties, which, despite their non.-commercial engagement in GAVI, nonetheless exist by their corporate definition to maximize profits. Whilst there may be clear technical roles that commercial partners can and need to play within GAVI, their involvement as a partner should not compromise the independence of GAVI's governance function.
>
> This observation is made particularly poignant in the light of the fact that three current members of the Board are engaged in the development or production of vaccines being promoted by GAVI: at the time of research, Aventis Pasteur of the DTPHepBHib vaccine, the Institut Pasteur of the yellow fever vaccine, and the Centre for Genetic Engineering and Biotechnology of the Hib vaccine.

The paper then recommended that GAVI re-examine its structure and separate the principle of partnership from that of governance by ensuring that mechanisms exist to avoid conflicts of interest. Until such analysis was undertaken, all commercial interests of Board members should be declared in a transparent manner. Commercial partners with a potential conflict of interest should not sit on the Board that governs the Alliance's strategic direction.

Conclusion

The aim of the $750 million Gates Foundation donation was to reach a 'simple' goal: to fulfill the right of every child to be protected against vaccine-preventable diseases of public health concern (Hardon, 2001).

Not a simple goal, but an ambitious and worthy objective which GAVI and other immunization schemes are trying to reach in spite of considerable obstacles. Some are common to all development efforts: failing or failed states, poor political governance, corruption, civil and external wars, failing economies, natural disasters. Some are specific to public health and immunization programmes: lack of political commitment to health programmes, weak state of health infrastructure, poorly trained health personnel, insufficient financial resources, unsafe injection practices, inadequate cold chain, shortages of vaccines.

On GAVI itself, concerns have been identified: too-rapid implementation; delayed vaccine supply; doubts about sustainability in view of the limited-time donation, unclear coordination between the multiple immunization initiatives.

On the positive side, the creation of the Alliance and of the Vaccine Fund have usefully renewed focus on immunization for industrialized and developing countries, and for the industry. It is expected that GAVI will provide a much needed stability to delivery systems, demand creation and vaccine supply. Dr Godal dismissed as 'complete nonsense' the allegations in the popular media that GAVI was creating profitable new outlets for vaccine manufacturers rather than preventing disease (Godal, 2002). He wrote that 'If the public sector can work to help make the developing-country vaccine environment more attractive to vaccine manufacturers, children living in the poorest countries will have access to better and more effective vaccines'. GAVI officials recognize that the Vaccine Fund cannot be the answer to all resource needs, but they stress that GAVI is acting as a catalyst for other sources of funding, including increases in national governments' own health budgets, other bilateral donor funding and development loans, or through mechanisms such as debt relief.

The participation of business partners in the GAVI Board and in the Board of the Vaccine Fund has been hailed as a way to effectively involve the vaccine industry in immunization programmes as equal partners with governments, international organizations, foundations and NGOs. The aim is to obtain their support and cooperation, their technical expertise, and to encourage the producers to lower their prices for the poor countries. National and international public health needs the vaccine industry for its capacity in research and development of new vaccines, its production of existing vaccines, its capacity to deliver vaccines.

Should industry representatives be 'equal partners' with WHO, and UNICEF? Can profit objectives be possibly merged into public health demands? Should there be limits to business participation in such schemes as GAVI? WHO, as the directing and coordinating authority on international health work, promotes 'Health For All', and the provision of accessible and affordable medicines and vaccines to all, with a focus on developing countries. The conditions set by an industry representative for its participation in the Alliance are due to clash with WHO's mandate and advocacy: the guarantee of 'reasonable prices' (what are reasonable prices?), respect for international property rights (patents) and a prohibition on Doha-approved compulsory licensing. The position of industry representatives in GAVI and the Vaccine Fund Boards may reveal conflicts of interest, unless full transparency is assured.

The recommendation of Save the Children UK that GAVI re-examined its structure and separate the principle of partnership from that of governance should be considered seriously. In the meantime, there is a need for strong control by the GAVI Executive Secretary, by the boards of WHO and UNICEF, and monitoring by the concerned NGOs.

While the international health organizations need to maintain good relations with the vaccine producers with a view to promoting production, research and development of vaccines against diseases of main concern to developing countries, external pressure by NGOs will remain essential to compel a reluctant industry to lower the prices of existing and new vaccines for those countries, as they are doing for AIDS medicines, and to allow these countries to develop their own industry.

Notes

1   The Global Advisory Group had been appointed to advise WHO on its EPI – see WHO Doc. WHO/EPI/GEN/94.1, 1994.
2   In 2003, the members of GAVI's Board included three developing country governments (Mongolia, Mozambique, India), three industrialized country governments (Canada, UK and USA), the US Centers for Disease Control and Prevention (CDC) as a technical health institute, the Sierra Leone Red Cross Society as an NGO, and the UN Foundation, in addition to business-related members.
3   The specific vaccine industry partners involved in GAVI are those that produce the greatest share of the global vaccine supply. They were, in 2002: Aventis Pasteur, SmithKline Beecham, American Home Products, Merck & Co., Inc., Chiron Vaccines, BERNA Swiss Serum & Vaccine Institute Berne (representing smaller vaccine producers).
4   Members of the Vaccine Fund's Board of Directors include several widely known and esteemed former politicians (Nelson Mandela, Graça Machel, Jacques Delors, Jens Stoltenberg), the Queen of Jordan, the President of the Vaccine Fund, Jacques-François Martin, the Executive Secretary of GAVI (Dr Tore Godal), the co-chair and President of the Bill & Melinda Gates Foundation, Mstislav Rostropovich, the cellist and defender of human rights, Mary Robinson, the former High Commissioner for Human Rights, the Chairman of the US Fund for UNICEF, the President of Harvard University, in addition to business-related members.

PART IV
FIGHTING THE INDUSTRY

Chapter 10

Tobacco, the Perfect 'Foe'

In her first statement to the World Health Assembly, on 13 May 1998, Dr Brundtland, newly elected Director-General of WHO stated bluntly: 'Tobacco is a killer'. In another statement, she added:

> Four million unnecessary deaths per year. It is rare – if not impossible – to find examples in history that match tobacco's programmed trail of destruction. I use the word programmed carefully. A cigarette is the only consumer product which when used as directed kills the consumer (WHO, 1998d).

She then launched the 'Tobacco Free Initiative' as one of her major priorities. Shortly before she left WHO, on 21 May 2003, the World Health Assembly adopted the WHO Framework Convention on Tobacco Control, perhaps the most impressive achievement of her five-year mandate.

In contrast with programmes described in previous Chapters, the fight against tobacco has not created a partnership with the industry. Parnerships with the pharmaceutical industry or with vaccine producers are necessary or desirable, under certain conditions, for the fight against AIDS or poliomyelitis. However, as the objective of tobacco control is to 'protect present and future generations from tobacco consumption and exposure to tobacco smoke', in the words of the Convention, through curbing consumption and exposure, all measures proposed or taken to control tobacco production and use are in direct conflict with the industry's objective of increasing profits through increased production, coverage and consumption. The revenues of the tobacco industry depend on the number of people addicted to smoking. Tobacco products have the capacity to cause addiction, due to their nicotine content and other substances in the emission. Manufacturing processes can further add to the toxicants and can make nicotine more readily available for absorption into the body, increasing the addictive effects of nicotine. The conflict between the tobacco industry and public health authorities has been compounded by the industry's hidden efforts to undermine or subvert tobacco control efforts at both national and international levels.

Statistics and scientific facts

Tobacco is estimated to account for just over 3 million annual deaths in 1990, rising to 4.023 million annual deaths in 1998. WHO estimates that deaths attributable to tobacco will rise to 8.4 million in 2020 and reach 10 million annual deaths in about 2030 (2003d). By 2020, tobacco use will cause 17.7 per cent of all deaths in developed countries, and 10.9 per cent of all deaths in developing countries. In most of the world, the harmful health effects of tobacco come from smoking cigarettes, either manufactured or hand rolled. Nevertheless, tobacco can have many of the same effects when consumed in various smokeless tobacco forms or when smoked in cigars.

The health impacts of tobacco are often described in the biomedical literature. A first wave of publications linked smoking with lung cancer around 1950 (Collin, Lee & Bissell, 2002:266). A Monograph on Tobacco Smoking issued in 1986 by the International Agency for Research on Cancer (IARC, 1986)[1] concluded in part that:

> There is sufficient evidence that tobacco smoke is carcinogenic to humans, – The occurrence of malignant tumors of the respiratory tract and of the upper digestive tract is causally related to the smoking of different forms of tobacco (cigarettes, cigars, pipes, *bidis*). The occurrence of malignant tumors of the bladder, renal pelvis and pancreas is causally related to the smoking of cigarettes.

Tobacco is the most important cause of lung cancer. It kills even more people through many other diseases, including cancers at other sites, heart disease, stroke, emphysema and other chronic lung diseases. On average, lifetime smokers have a 50 per cent chance of dying from tobacco. Half of these will die in middle age, before age 70, losing 22 years of normal life expectancy in developed countries. In 1990, smoking was responsible for 35 per cent of all male deaths occurring in middle age (age 35–69) in these countries (WHO, 1997b).

Environmental tobacco smoke (ETS) contains essentially all of the same carcinogens and toxic agents that are inhaled by the smoker. ETS is harmful to non-smokers because it causes lung cancer and other diseases and aggravates allergies and asthma. Maternal smoking is associated with a higher risk of miscarriage, lower birth-weight of babies, and inhibited child development. Parental smoking is also a factor in sudden infant death syndrome and is associated with higher rates of respiratory illnesses, including bronchitis, colds, and pneumonia in children.

Besides being a serious public health problem, tobacco use is also a major drain on the world's financial resources and a major threat to sustainable and equitable development. A World Bank study entitled 'The Economic Costs and Benefits of Investing in Tobacco' (March 1993) has estimated that the use of tobacco results in a global net loss of $200 billion per year, with half of these losses occurring in developing countries. The study estimated that smoking prevention is among the most cost-effective of all health interventions (WHO, 1997c).

In a study commissioned by Philip Morris, carried out by the consulting firm Arthur D. Little in 2001, the many 'positive' economic effects of smoking include 'health care cost savings due to early mortality'. While confirming the lethal effect of smoking, the report showed a brazen and unethical disregard of the value of human life itself (Herbert, 2001).

National and international control measures

Reducing the tobacco epidemic requires a comprehensive approach based on scientific evidence, including government, community and media action, health education, and legislative measures. Tobacco control efforts are necessary at local, national and international levels, in a complementary fashion.

The central role of governments

In many cases, national programmes and policies have come about because of efforts begun at the local level, often initiated by grassroot organizations or committed individuals.

However, governments retain a central and crucial role in tobacco control, as they do in most public health programmes. Without government commitment, tobacco control measures are less likely to succeed. Based on World Health Assembly resolutions, WHO has defined a 'Ten-Point Programme for Successful Tobacco Control': see Presentation 10.1.

Presentation 10.1

WHO's Ten-Point Programme for Successful Tobacco Control

1. Protection for children from becoming addicted to tobacco through such measures as the banning of sales to and advertising targeted at children.
2. Implementation of fiscal policies to discourage the use of tobacco, such as tobacco taxes that increase faster than the growth in prices and income.
3. Allocation of a portion of the money raised from tobacco taxes to finance other tobacco control and health promotion measures.
4. Health promotion, health education and smoking cessation programmes. Health workers and institutions set an example by being smoke-free.
5. Protection from involuntary exposure to environmental tobacco smoke (ETS).
6. Elimination of socioeconomic, behavioural and other incentives which maintain and promote the use of tobacco.
7. Elimination of direct and indirect tobacco advertising, promotion and sponsorship.
8. Controls on tobacco products, including prominent health warnings on tobacco products and in any remaining advertisements; limits on and mandatory reporting of toxic constituents in tobacco products and tobacco smoke.
9. Promotion of economic alternatives to tobacco growing and manufacturing.
10. Effective management, monitoring and evaluation of tobacco issues.

Source: WHO *Fact-Sheet* No. 159, May 1997.

WHO notes that government action has been remarkably uneven on tobacco control in marked contrast to the relatively constant effective public health response to such issues as immunization (WHO, 1997d). Convincing smokers to stop smoking, and increasing the price of cigarettes is less 'sexy' than vaccinating young children against polio. The long delay between smoking and the diseases it causes may cause denial by smokers, inhibiting their motivation to stop smoking. Also, the interest of vaccine producers is to increase their sales by promoting immunization, while anti-tobacco campaigns aim at reducing tobacco production, marketing and use; thus reducing sales and profits.

Some governments may reject tobacco control in order to protect their private tobacco producers; or their state tobacco monopoly, some may fear a loss of state revenues due to less sales of tobacco products; some may not be fully aware of, or believe in, the health and economic consequences of tobacco use; some are more open to pressures from the tobacco industry. All governments and populations are exposed to the industry's overt or covert campaigns, denying tobacco's dangerous effects on health and asserting its 'good conduct'. Smokers may resist anti-tobacco laws and their implementation.

As reported by WHO in 1996, in the early 1990s, about 25 countries had laws that prohibited the sale of cigarettes to minors, with the age of prohibition ranging from 16 to 21 years of age (WHO, 1996b). In some cases, other related measures were enacted, including bans or restrictions on cigarette sales from vending machines, prohibitions on sales of tobacco products and smoking in schools, prohibiting the sale of single cigarettes and banning the offering of free samples of cigarettes. Many jurisdictions have laws that ban or restrict smoking in public places, workplaces and transit vehicles.

Also in the early 1990s, about 80 countries required health warnings to appear on packages of tobacco products. However, in most of these countries, the warnings were small, inconspicuous and provided little information about the serious health consequences of tobacco use. By the mid-1990s, however, a number of countries had adopted more stringent warning systems, involving direct statements of health hazards, multiple messages, as well as large and prominent display. A number of countries have passed law to ban all or nearly all forms of tobacco advertising. In a number of countries, further government or legislative action was required in order to tighten advertising restrictions, as tobacco companies had attempted to circumvent bans by the use of indirect advertising.

As of the mid-1990s, Finland, Iceland, Norway, Portugal and Singapore had long-standing comprehensive tobacco control policies, built up gradually since the 1970s. Other countries, such as Australia, France, New Zealand, Sweden and Thailand have more recently implemented programmes encompassing elements called by World Health Assembly resolutions.

An effective national tobacco control policy requires legislation action, whether in the form of adopting or amending laws, regulation or government decrees. However, as shown in the following example, ineffective enforcement may render the legislation ineffective. In France, government commitment and the adoption of a law stumbled over smokers' resistance to change, and the lack of enforcement by state authorities of compliance with the law by private and public institutions.

France and tobacco

France has been slow in fighting tobacco use, in order to protect its own state industry and brand (the infamous 'Gauloises'). Its state business interests have long prevailed over health concerns. The first anti-tobacco (and anti-alcohol) law, the 'Loi Evin', was adopted on 10 January 1991. It prohibited all direct or indirect promotion of tobacco, set maximum tar contents of cigarettes, imposed label warnings on tobacco products that they cause 'serious harm to health', requested that cigarette packages showed their average content of tar and nicotine. The law forbade smoking in public, collective places, in particular in schools, and in collective transport, except in places reserved for smokers. A 'Day without tobacco' was to be set.

The law was not properly enforced. Many private and public cafés and restaurants ignored it and were not sanctioned. Some progress was noted: eight per cent less tobacco was smoked between 1991 and 1996, a decrease due in part to the law and price increases – 93 billion cigarettes sold in 1993, 83 billion in 1997.

The problem remains serious. In 1998, 60,000 deaths were due to tobacco (56,000 men and 4,000 women). It was estimated that, by 2025, male mortality due to tobacco would double while female mortality would be multiplied by ten.[2] In 2003, the government ordered more price increases and Parliament forbade sales of tobacco products to minors (less than 16 years of age).

These new measures, which should be accompanied by an effective health education campaign and exemplary sanctions, should reduce more significantly the use of tobacco in France over the next few years.

International tobacco control

From 1970 to 1995, the World Health Assembly adopted 14 resolutions, all without dissent, in favour of tobacco control measures. Several of these resolutions called for comprehensive tobacco control programmes and policies.

In 1995, Dr Hiroshi Nakajima, Dr Brundtland's predecessor as WHO Director-General, blamed publicly the tobacco industry's greed for the tobacco epidemic or pandemic (Nakajima, 1995): 'The world over, tobacco manufacturers and merchants put their own financial interests before the health and lives of the thousand million consumers to whom they sell their products ... tobacco kills'. As tobacco is a commodity in international trade, he stated that the fight against tobacco must be worldwide, based on a concerted global strategy.

In the 1990s, the World Bank stopped granting loans for projects linked to the growing or manufacture of tobacco. The International Civil Aviation Organization adopted a resolution calling for a ban on smoking on all international flights by 1 January 1996. Several UN agencies provide their staff with a smoke-free environment.

The WHO Regional Office for the Western Pacific instituted the Action Plan on Tobacco or Health for 1995–1999. The Plan called for a tobacco-advertising free region by the year 2000, a percentage of tobacco tax to be allocated to fund sports, arts and health promotion, all airlines to be smoke-free, all countries to cut or reduce consumption and all countries to prevent a rise in smoking among women (WHO, 1997e).

In May 1996, the World Health Assembly requested the Director-General to initiate the development of a framework convention in accordance with Article 19 of the WHO Constitution. On 28 May 1997, World No-Tobacco Day 1997, Dr Nakajima called upon governments, organizations and individuals around the world to work together for a tobacco-free world and finally say to the tobacco industry 'enough is enough' (WHO, 1997f).

One year later, Dr Brundtland, the new Director-General, chose the fight against tobacco as one of her major priorities. In October 1998, she nominated Dr Derek Yach as Programme Manager of the Tobacco Free Initiative at WHO headquarters in Geneva. In January 1999, at the Davos World Economic Forum, Dr Brundtland announced the creation of the WHO European Partnership Project on Tobacco Dependence, open to both private, non-commercial and public sector partners. It included three major pharmaceutical companies, Glaxo Wellcome, Novartis Consumer Health and Pharmacia & Upjohn, all manufacturers of treatment products for tobacco dependence. It is noteworthy that this project was presented by WHO as a model which could provide a basis for future partnerships with the private sector in other important health areas (WHO, 1999i).

WHO went one step further in its fight against tobacco when the organization called on international food and drug regulators to bring cigarettes and other tobacco industry products under the same ambit of rules that govern the sales and promotion of other nicotine delivery products. On 26 April 1999, Dr Brundtland declared: 'A cigarette is a euphemism for a cleverly crafted product that delivers just the right amount of nicotine to keep its user addicted for life before killing the person'. For tobacco control experts, it does not stand to reason that harmful nicotine from cigarettes is available freely while prescriptions are necessary for therapeutic nicotine sold by pharmaceutical companies. Food sold by tobacco companies is regulated but their cigarettes brands are not. In 1890, tobacco was included in the US Pharmacopia but, after intense lobbying of Congress by tobacco manufacturers, it was excluded from the purview of the US Food and Drug Administration, which was created in 1906 with jurisdiction over those products listed in Pharmacopia (WHO, 1999j). WHO's demand is however unlikely to be met.

In May 1999, the World Health Assembly established an Intergovernmental Negotiating Body, open to all Member States, to draft and negotiate the proposed WHO Framework Convention on Tobacco Control (Res. WHA52.18 – see below).

Continuing its verbal attacks, and not mincing its words, WHO launched another campaign in November 1999 to counter tobacco industry 'deception' around the world. Called 'Tobacco Kills Don't Be Duped', the campaign brought together senior health and media activists from 20 countries to join forces with Dr Jeffrey Wigand, the tobacco industry whistle-blower, and California's successful anti-smoking programme to expose big tobacco's worldwide campaign of deceptions and lies. Dr Brundtland called tobacco a communicated disease (by reference to communicable diseases) – communicated through advertising. The WHO campaign was to strengthen the ability of broadcast and newspaper journalists, and other health communicators worldwide to sift facts from fiction about tobacco use, its spread and promotion (WHO, 1999k).

Also in November 1999, WHO organized an International Conference on Tobacco and Health in Kobe (Japan), on 'Avoiding the Tobacco Epidemic in Women and Youth'. It brought together close to 500 of Asia's top public health experts and anti-tobacco campaigners. The number of adolescent and young adult women smoking in Japan had increased alarmingly in recent years and other Asian countries could soon experience the same phenomenon if action was not taken to prevent the epidemic from spreading. The 'Kobe Declaration' demanded that the proposed Framework Convention on Tobacco Control (FCTC) should 'include gender-specific concerns and perspectives in each and every aspect' and states that 'gender equality in society must be an integral part of tobacco control strategies and women's leadership is essential to success'.

In July 2000, the Committee of Experts on Tobacco Industry Documents, appointed by WHO, submitted its report on 'Tobacco Company Strategies to Undermine Tobacco Control Activities' (called 'Experts Report' hereunder)(WHO, 2000a). It described in detail the use by tobacco companies of 'unacceptable strategies and tactics' (see below). In May 2001, the World Health Assembly noted with great concern the findings of the Committee of Experts, namely that the tobacco industry had operated for years with the expressed intention of subverting the role of governments and of WHO in implementing public health policies to combat the tobacco epidemic. It urged Member States to be aware of affiliations between the tobacco industry and members of their delegations. It recognized that public confidence would be enhanced by transparency of affiliation between delegates to the Health Assembly and other meetings of WHO and the tobacco industry.

In January 2002, the WHO Executive Board admitted into official relations with the Organization the International Non Governmental Coalition Against Tobacco and *Infact* (Res. ED109.R22). Since 1977, *Infact* has worked internationally to advance public health in the face of powerful corporate interests. The NGO contributed forcefully to the adoption of the WHO's International Code of Marketing Breast-Milk Substitutes in 1981.

The Framework Convention on Tobacco Control was adopted unanimously by the World Health Assembly on 21 May 2003 (Res. WHA56.1). It was the first international treaty negotiated under the auspices of WHO. The Convention was open for signature by States on 16 June 2003.

The tobacco companies' strategies

These strategies are amply and convincingly described in the Experts Report. In the summer of 1999, an internal report to the Director-General of WHO suggested that there was evidence in formerly confidential tobacco company documents[3] that these companies had made 'efforts to prevent implementation of healthy public policy and efforts to reduce funding of tobacco control within UN organizations'. Responding to this report, Dr Brundtland assembled a Committee of four independent experts[4] to research the once confidential, now publicly available, tobacco company documents.

According to the Report's Foreword:

The tobacco companies' own documents[5] show that they viewed WHO, an international public health agency, as one of their foremost enemies. The documents show further that the tobacco companies instigated global strategies to discredit and impede WHO's ability to carry out its mission. The tobacco companies' campaign against WHO was rarely directed at the merits of the public health issues raised by tobacco use. Instead, the documents show that tobacco companies sought to divert attention from the public health issues, to reduce budgets for the scientific and policy activities carried out by WHO, to pit other UN agencies against WHO, to convince developing countries that WHO's tobacco control programme was a 'First World' agenda carried out at the expense of the developing world, to distort the results of important scientific studies on tobacco, and to discredit WHO as an institution.

Although these strategies and tactics were frequently devised at the highest levels of tobacco companies, the role of tobacco industry officials in carrying out these strategies was often concealed. In their campaign against WHO, the documents show that tobacco companies hid behind a variety of ostensibly independent quasi-academic, public policy, and business organizations whose tobacco industry funding was not disclosed. The documents also show that tobacco company strategies to undermine WHO relied heavily on international and scientific experts with hidden financial ties to the industry. Perhaps most disturbing, the documents show that tobacco companies quietly influenced other UN agencies and representatives of developing countries to resist WHO's tobacco control initiatives.

... it is reasonable to believe that the tobacco companies' subversion of WHO's tobacco control activities has resulted in significant harm ...

In order to influence WHO's tobacco control activities, tobacco companies maintained and developed relationships with current or former WHO staff, consultants and advisers. In some cases, the companies hired or offered future employment to former WHO or UN officials. The companies also had their own consultants in positions in WHO, paying them to serve their interests while working for WHO.

Tobacco company lobbying was aimed at influencing FAO, a 'natural ally', to take a stance against WHO's tobacco control policies by promoting the economic importance of tobacco as more significant that the health consequences of tobacco use. The companies also targeted the World Bank, the UN Conference on Trade and Development (UNCTAD), the UN Economic and Social Council (ECOSOC) and the ILO. In order to 'redirect WHO', Philip Morris used its own food companies and other non-tobacco subsidiaries, as well as tobacco industry organizations, business organizations, front groups and other ostensibly independent surrogates. Philip Morris pressed business groups such as the International Chamber of Commerce to lobby the World Health Assembly.

According to the Experts Report, tobacco company documents suggest that Paul Dietrich, an American lawyer with long-term ties to tobacco companies, played a significant role in the companies' strategy of undermining WHO's tobacco control activities. He wrote articles and editorials attacking WHO's priorities, which were published in major media outlets. He gave presentations to journalists and government officials on WHO's inappropriate spending. No mention was ever made in his articles and presentations that he received significant tobacco company funding. The documents indicate that Dietrich attempted to redirect the priorities of the Pan American Health Organization (PAHO) away from tobacco, when he was appointed to PAHO's Development Committee. PAHO also serves as WHO's Regional Office for the Americas. PAHO and Dietrich have rejected the account provided by the documents. However, the Experts Committee believed that there are significant conflict of interest issues raised by holding a position on a PAHO committee while simultaneously working for the tobacco industry. The Committee made recommendations to help ensure that such conflicts do not arise in the future.

Targeting the International Agency for Research on Cancer (IARC)

In April 2000, *The Lancet* described the tobacco industry efforts to subvert a large scale epidemiological study on the relationship between environmental tobacco smoke (ETS) and lung cancer (Ong, Glantz, 2000). The study was conducted by the WHO-affiliated International Agency for Research on Cancer (IARC).

Initiated in 1988, the IARC ETS study was an international, collaborative case-control study to assess the relationship between exposure to ETS and other environmental risk factors and the risk of lung cancer in subjects who had never smoked tobacco. In 1993, Philip Morris launched a wide-ranging, well-funded campaign to influence the conduct of the study and the interpretation of the results. The IARC study cost $2 million over ten years. Philip Morris planned to spend $2 million in one year alone and up to $4 million on research.

The Expert Report found that tobacco companies successfully concealed their role in establishing contacts with the IARC investigators, and funded and publicized research designed to cast doubt on the validity of the IARC study. Through their contacts with IARC investigators and collaborators, tobacco companies gained a great deal of information about the design, conduct, and analysis of the study, as well as information on preliminary results. Some of this information was intended to be kept confidential. The tobacco companies' communication strategy was the most successful (and destructive) element of its attempt to undermine IARC's study. By distorting the statistical underpinnings of the study results, tobacco industry officials managed to convince journalists around the world to write news stories that the study showed no increased risk of lung cancer from ETS exposure in non-smokers.

Ultimately, however, the tobacco industry's efforts to influence the methodology of the study did not appear to have altered the study results or analysis, one of their objectives. In spite of the industry's insidious campaign, IARC released its Monograph on Tobacco Smoking and Smoke in 2002 (IARC, 2002). The study concluded that tobacco smoking and tobacco smoke are carcinogenic to humans.

The Experts Report recommended that WHO rules be strengthened by screening prospective employees, consultants, advisors, and committee members for conflicts of interest, and clarifying the consequences of violations of ethical rules. In conclusion, the Experts' inquiry demonstrated that tobacco is unlike other threats to health: 'Reversing the epidemic of tobacco use will be about more than fighting addiction and disease; it will be about overcoming a determined and powerful industry, many of whose most important counter-strategies are carried out in secret'.

The Framework Convention on Tobacco Control

The negotiations leading to the adoption of the Convention recalled those which preceded the adoption of the International Code of Marketing of Breast-milk Substitutes in 1981, with a few differences (see Chapter 3).

The legal form of the two instruments is different: the Code was adopted as a non-binding recommendation under Article 23 of the WHO Constitution, while the Convention has been adopted as a binding international treaty under Article 19 of the Constitution. This was the first time that WHO has exercised its constitutional mandate to negotiate and approve a binding Convention.

The actors were the same: governments favourable or hostile to the proposed instrument, NGOs promoting a solid text, multinational companies trying to limit the scope of the instrument, WHO, as the representative of international public health. However, WHO's position was different in the negotiations for the Code and for the Convention. WHO took sides as a strong supporter of the future Convention; in opposition to the tobacco industry, with full support of the NGOs, while the Organization tried to remain an intermediary between the industry and NGOs in order to obtain a consensus on the Code. As another difference, the baby food enterprises are not the enemy of WHO, as is the tobacco industry, although both are profit-driven and tried to stop or water down the Code and the Convention.

Why an international Convention? Production and sales of tobacco products remain largely within the regulatory control of governments. However, the open or hidden power of the tobacco industry vs. governments, particularly in the developing world, in targeting selected populations within and across countries through marketing, advertising and sponsorship, has the potential to circumvent national regulatory authority. Governments may benefit from clear and binding policies defined on scientifically sound bases and agreed at the international level, in order to resist multinational companies' enticements. The development of the Convention was expected to encourage Member States to strengthen their own national tobacco control policies. The negotiating process was also expected to mobilize national and international technical and financial support for tobacco control, raise global awareness about the unnecessary burden of disease brought about by tobacco use and expose the tobacco industry's practices.

Governments: for or against?

While the Convention was adopted unanimously on 21 May 2003 by all WHO Member States, this final unanimity came only after strong oppositions and divergences from a few countries were overcome or papered over during the negotiations.

Most countries in Africa, the Middle East and Southeast Asia were in favour of a strong Convention. However, Malawi under the influence of its tobacco growers' interests, spoke against a strong Convention.

Brazil, supported by Latin American countries, was perceived as somewhat lenient to Big Tobacco. The Brazilian chairmen of the negotiations were accused by health activists of having weakened drafts of the Convention. The last Chairman, Luiz Felipe de Seixas Correa replied that his aim was to arrive at an 'effective' treaty: 'The task of the negotiations is to bridge the gap between what is desirable and what is possible', he told journalists (AP, 2003).

Both Japan and China had officials of their Tobacco State Monopoly in their delegations to the negotiations. Japan's government is the majority shareholder in the world's third largest tobacco transnational. An official report from Japan's Fiscal System Council acknowledged tobacco's health risks but characterized them as luxury items that should not be phased out. The report opposed banning words like 'mild' and 'light' on labels (which were banned by the Convention), saying that the words describe the taste, not the products' impact on health (UN Foundation, 2002).

The European Union gave support to the future Convention in the negotiations, although Germany was initially seen as a strong and consistent ally of the tobacco industry. In June 2003, Mr David Byrnes, EU Commissioner for Health and Consumer Protection, received the WHO Director-General's Award for leadership in global tobacco control, and in supporting the establishment of an effective and comprehensive Convention.

During the negotiations, the US placed itself in an ambiguous position. One of the countries with the most stringent anti-tobacco rules, it was generally described as openly intent on weakening the text of the future Convention, in reflecting the positions of the tobacco industry. On 12 October 2002, the head of the US delegation to the negotiating conference, the Deputy Assistant Secretary for Health Tom Novotny, said: 'As an international leader in tobacco control, we are prepared to negotiate a strong agreement among nations to take coordinated, effective steps to drastically improve global health by decreasing tobacco use' (US Mission, 2000). These words were contradicted by the interventions of the US negotiators during the sessions, which drove all efforts to the lowest common denominator.

When the last negotiations concluded on 1 March 2003, the US delegate told a plenary session that the US had reservations about several clauses and that it would be exploring options to have the treaty changed. In a last minute effort to weaken the Convention, the US sent a letter to WHO and to the Health Ministers of all WHO Member States in April 2003 proposing to introduce a 'reservations' clause, which would allow governments to opt out of any provision which they find objectionable. The final text of the Convention does not allow such reservations. On 18 May, another US delegate, the Secretary of Health and Human Services Tommy Thompson, said that the US would not seek any changes in the treaty and would adopt it (Langley, 2003a).

The US opposition to a binding Convention may be explained, albeit not justified, by its general reluctance to enter into international commitments, compounded by the Bush administration's rejection of several international treaties. This position may be based on the US will to protect its freedom of decision and its national sovereignty, and on legal constitutional grounds such as the federal nature of the US and states' rights. Another less admissible reason, often invoked by NGOs, is the excessive influence of the tobacco industry on the Bush administration. Whatever the reasons, the difference between US domestic policies and the position it takes at the international level remains striking.

The NGOs for a strong Convention

NGO groups, including the Network for Accountability of the Tobacco Transnationals (NATT) and the Framework Convention Alliance, built support for including strong corporate accountability measures in the Convention. During the negotiation sessions, they lobbied WHO officials, national delegates and issued statements denouncing the motives and practices of the tobacco companies.

Infact[6] developed the following principles with input from other organizations and experts for the treaty to realize the potential to reverse the tobacco addiction pandemic. Excerpts:

- Non-state actors with tobacco interests disqualify themselves from lobbying on legislation related to tobacco and health. They must disclose all other lobbying expenditures and political contributions. State actors should refuse contributions from tobacco interests. A transparency of affiliation should exist between government officials and tobacco interests;
- As a result of the addictive and harmful nature of tobacco products, normal trade practices are not applicable. Exclude tobacco as a trade item in bilateral and multilateral agreements;
- Tobacco corporations should be held accountable for past, present and future harm, including but not limited to legal processes;
- States shall support and/or initiate the economic conversion from tobacco agriculture, production, and promotion to healthier and more environmentally sustainable alternatives;
- States, particularly those that charter the tobacco transnational corporation, and international bodies should monitor the national and transnational activities of the tobacco corporations, including advertising and promotion, political contributions and lobbying, joint ventures, acquisitions, revenues and profits, possible links to smuggling activities, interference in public health policy, and misrepresentation of the addictive nature and hazardous health effects of tobacco.

The tobacco industry: for a weak Convention

The industry used several strategies to fight against a binding Convention. Its influence was directly applied through having representatives of tobacco industry trade associations serving in countries' delegations (*Infact*, 2003) . For instance, the Chief Executive for the International Tobacco Growers Association of Africa and the General Manager of the Tobacco Exporters Association of Malawi served on Malawi's delegation at the fifth session of the negotiation (INB5). Other countries also had delegates closely tied to the tobacco industry. At the same session, China sent two officials of its State Tobacco Monopoly, and Turkey the Deputy Director-General of its State Monopoly. Japan had five members of its Ministry of Finance, which owns a 67 per cent stake in Japan Tobacco.

At the same session, British American Tobacco (BAT) had at least twelve representatives. Also attending were the Chief Executive of the International Tobacco Growers Association worldwide, the Director General of the International

Travel Retail Confederation and representatives of the International Association of Airport Duty Free Stores, with links to the tobacco industry.

WHO released in 2002 internal *Japan Tobacco International* (JTI) documents of October 2001 detailing strategies to fight the Convention (*Infact*, 2002). As defined by a British tobacco consultant, Roger Scruton, they included:

- A suggestion to 'shift the onus back on to the WHO to justify the vindictiveness of its attack', with 'more explicit mention of other products that are open to the same criticisms as tobacco and which ought to be of equal concern to the WHO'. Scruton proposed to divert the WHO's energy from tobacco by drawing attention to the harmful effects of fast food and alcohol.
- A plan to place 'articles in the influential media, whose effect will be to discredit the FCTC process'. Questions to be planted with the press include, 'why is tobacco being singled out ...?' and 'why is a global treaty necessary ...?'
- A strategy to reframe the issue 'as one of freedom of choice', urging 'responsible choice' into the Convention.

Scruton presented the Convention's general obligations as a 'threat to national sovereignty'. The US, China and Pakistan used this argument during the negotiations.

The proposals for 2002 included regular meetings over lunch or dinner between JTI personnel and key persons for informal discussions, use of media contacts to place relevant articles on such topics as 'mendacious campaigns against the industry', ' use of tobacco legislation as a diversionary tactic in times of rising moral corruption '[!], the Convention described as 'an attempt to police the lifestyles of ordinary people, by an institution which is entirely unaccountable to them'.

Another strategy was to promote a Code of Conduct in an attempt to pre-empt the negotiations for a convention, a strategy previously used by the infant food producers during the negotiations for the International Code of Marketing of Breast-Milk Substitutes. On 10 September 2001, eleven months after the start of the Convention negotiations, British American Tobacco, Philip Morris, and Japan Tobacco announced a new code of conduct on international marketing standards, ostensibly to prevent sales activities being targeted at non-smokers and young people (Kapp, 2001a). The standards, due to come into force early 2003, would eliminate sponsorship of big sporting events, advertisements on the internet, television and radio, celebrity endorsements, advertisements suggesting that smoking enhances athletic, professional or sexual success and advertisements aimed at or appealing to youth.

Dr Brundtland replied: 'We see no evidence that tobacco companies are capable of self-regulation'. According to WHO, 'Voluntary codes of advertising were first adopted – and found wanting – by the US, Canada and the UK'. Independent research published by Credit Suisse First Boston found that the elimination of certain marketing activities was unlikely to decrease overall advertising. Many developed countries already had stricter legislation than the proposed standards. Health activists and WHO warned that the proposed voluntary controls were merely an attempt to derail the framework Convention.

The negotiation and adoption of the Convention

In May 1999, the World Health Assembly established an Intergovernmental Negotiating Body, open to all Member States, to draft and negotiate the proposed Convention and possible related protocols (Res. WHA52.18).

The first session of the Negotiating Body, held on 16–21 October 2000 in Geneva, was attended by representatives of 148 Member States, observers from the European Union, nine other intergovernmental organizations, and 25 NGOs. The session was preceded by two days of public hearings. WHO received 514 written submissions. During the hearings, testimonies were given by representatives of 144 private sector and non-governmental organizations and institutions, covering all regions of the world.

Not surprisingly, the hearings highlighted the key differences between the position of tobacco companies and related bodies, and public health institutions on the role of taxes of tobacco products; the risk of environmental tobacco smoke and passive smoking; and the contribution of advertising to smoking, especially among youth. Most tobacco companies questioned whether the convention could be a single global regulation, citing national sovereignty, the appropriateness of regulation at the national level, and self-regulation. Representatives of public health institutions on the other hand strongly argued that a truly viable tobacco control had to be global in reach, while respecting country and culture-specific solutions (WHO, 2001n).

More differences emerged in the second session of 30 April–5 May 2001. NGO representatives said that the text drawn up by the Chairman of the Negotiating Body, Celso Amorim (Brazil) was too weak. The Convention risked being further watered down during the negotiations. The UK Director of Action on Smoking and Health (ASH), said: 'We expect the US to oppose any serious advertising restrictions, we expect the European Union to be weak on smuggling, and we expect Japan to try to block consumer protection measures like a ban on misleading "light" [low tar] branding' (Kapp, 2001b).

Further sessions ended with the sixth round in February 2003. NGOs again warned against the danger in making too many concessions, in an effort to find consensus among all Member States.

On 1 March 2003, the 171 Member States of WHO transmitted to the World Health Assembly for adoption the final text of the Framework Convention on Tobacco Control. However, a few countries, including the US and Germany, said that they would not adopt the Convention in its current form. The US delegate said that the wording in some sections either violated the US Constitution or was otherwise unacceptable. While the US did not object to forwarding the draft Convention to the Assembly, these issues would have to be addressed (Langley, 2003b).

The World Health Assembly adopted the Convention on 21 May 2003 (Res. WHA5 and Annex). The US had dropped its opposition and voted for the treaty. On 16 June, 27 Member States and the European Union signed the Convention. The Convention will enter into force after ratification by 40 countries. The US and China made no immediate commitment to sign it.

The Convention

In its Preamble, the Parties reflected the concern of the international community about the devastating worldwide health, social, economic and environmental consequences of tobacco consumption and exposure to tobacco smoke. They recognized that scientific evidence has unequivocally established that tobacco consumption and exposure to tobacco smoke cause death, disease and disability, and that there is a time lag between the exposure to smoking and the other uses of tobacco products and the onset of tobacco-related diseases. They also recognized that cigarettes and other tobacco products are highly engineered so as to create and maintain dependence. They recognized the need to be alert to any efforts by the tobacco industry to undermine or subvert tobacco control efforts and the need to be informed of activities of the tobacco industry that have a negative impact on tobacco control efforts.

Some of the important principles and obligations are listed hereunder:

Art. 4.1: Every person should be informed of the health consequences, addictive nature and mortal threat posed by tobacco consumption and exposure to tobacco smoke and effective legislative, executive, administrative or other measures should be contemplated at the appropriate government level to protect all persons from exposure to tobacco smoke.

Art. 4.4: Comprehensive multisectoral measures and responses to reduce consumption of all tobacco products at the national, regional and international levels are essential so as to prevent, in accordance with public health principles, the incidence of diseases, premature disability and mortality due to tobacco consumption and exposure to tobacco smoke.

In Article 6.1, the Parties recognize that price and tax measures are an effective and important means of reducing tobacco consumption by various segments of the population, in particular young persons.

Under Article 11.1, measures should be taken under national law to ensure that tobacco product packaging and labelling do not promote a tobacco product by any means that are false, misleading, deceptive or likely to create an erroneous impression that a particular tobacco product is less harmful than others, including terms such as 'low-tar', 'light', 'ultra-light', or 'mild'. Each package should include health warnings and messages, which should be 50 per cent or more of the principal display areas, but not less that 30 per cent.

Art. 12 refers to education, communication, training and public awareness.

Under Art. 13, Parties recognize that a comprehensive ban on advertising, promotion and sponsorship would reduce the consumption of tobacco products. Subject to a State's constitutional principles, each Party shall undertake a comprehensive ban of all tobacco advertising, promotion and sponsorship.

Art. 14 provides that Parties shall take effective measures to promote cessation of tobacco use and adequate treatment of tobacco dependence.

Under Art. 16, measures should prohibit the sales of tobacco products to persons under the age set by domestic law, national law or eighteen.

Under Art. 17, Parties shall promote economically viable alternatives for tobacco workers, growers, and individual sellers.

Other Articles refer to the protection of the environment, criminal and civil liability including compensation, scientific and technical cooperation and communication of information.

Under Article 30, no reservations may be made to the Convention.

Conclusion

The need and usefulness of public-private partnerships in public health have been demonstrated in previous Chapters, subject to various conditions. Tobacco control, as a counter example, shows that, at both the national and international levels, partnership with the tobacco industry is neither desirable nor possible, first in view of tobacco's demonstrated danger for public health, and secondly because of its constant campaigns of 'lies and deception' addressed to the general public, but also to governments, WHO and other health institutions. The industry has declared that WHO was its enemy and tried to de-stabilize its programmes, to infiltrate and influence its secretariat and committees. The tobacco industry has reincarnated the image of the 'evil' transnational corporation previously denounced and attacked by the activist NGOs in other areas.

WHO uncovered the industry's manoeuvers, mainly thanks to a paper trail revealed by US litigation and rightly fought back, with the support of 'like-minded' governments and NGOs, declaring tobacco control one of its major priorities. In the fight against tobacco, WHO changed its role: from its traditional role as a benevolent world health leader or partner, setting standards and preaching public health, it moved into the position of an aggressed and aggressive leader openly fighting against a devious, unprincipled, enemy. Tobacco control is the unique example of a programme in which WHO decided to wage war against an industry.

During the negotiations leading to the Convention, some governments played an ambiguous role, encouraged by 'big tobacco' to protect their tobacco growers and enterprises, their state monopolies, while also responding to the international public health movement for effective tobacco control and concerned about their international image.

The final adoption of the Convention is not the end of the battle. 40 ratifications are needed to allow the Convention to take effect. Then, national legislations will have to be checked and possibly revised in order to ensure their compatibility with the Convention. Then, governments will have to implement the new measures, under international monitoring by WHO and NGOs.

On 4 August 2003, the newly-elected Director-General of WHO, Dr Jong-wook Lee, urged countries to sign and ratify the Convention as quickly as possible to prevent further loss of lives from tobacco-related diseases. Stressing that the Convention's obligations were not the optimum, he encouraged countries to consider measures beyond those required by the Convention (WHO, 2003e).

As noted by analysts (Collin, Lee & Bissell, 2002:279), 'Regardless of the validity of on-going debates concerning the value of public-private partnerships for health, the politics of tobacco remain an important exception'. There is a fundamental incompatibility between public health and the objectives of the tobacco industry.

Notes

1 IARC is an autonomous agency of WHO established in Lyon (France). The IARC Monographs series publishes authoritative independent assessments by international experts of the carcinogenic risks posed to humans by a variety of agents, mixtures and exposures. IARC Monographs are well-known for their thoroughness, accuracy and integrity.

2 'Situation du tabagisme en France', http://www.sante.gouv.fr/htm/pointsurtabac/5tab11.htm, accessed on 16 July 2003.

3 The millions of pages of confidential tobacco company documents were made public as a result of lawsuits against the tobacco industry filed in the USA and the 1998 settlement agreement between the tobacco companies and most US States.

4 Thomas Zeltner, M.D., David A Kessler, M.D., Anke Martiny, Ph.D., Fazel Randera, M.D. This section summarizes or reproduces selected excerpts from the Experts Report.

5 The available documents came from Philip Morris Companies, Inc., R.J. Reynolds Tobacco Company, Brown & Williamson Tobacco Company, American Tobacco Company, Lorillard Tobacco Company, The Tobacco Institute, the Council for Tobacco Research and the British American Tobacco Company.

6 *Infact* was a founding member of the Network for Accountability of the Tobacco Transnationals (NATT), 65 organizations from 40 countries.

Conclusion

The interaction of WHO and other public health institutions with the private sector has vastly increased since the 1990s. During Dr Brundtland's mandate, from 1998 to 2003, WHO has openly and actively engaged into a number of alliances and partnerships with other IGOs, foundations, NGOs and for-profit enterprises. The new Director-General, Dr Lee Jong-wook, who took office on 21 July 2003, said in an interview that he was hoping that WHO would continue public-private cooperation. For example, he said that developing new diagnostic tools, finding new TB drugs, a malaria vaccine, could only be done through private-public, rich country-poor country partnerships (Newsweek, 2003).

This 'opening to business' of international health organizations, on lines similar to the UN Global Compact, has been developed within the context of globalization. At the national level, the role of the state was being re-assessed, in the belief that some of its functions might be better and more economically assumed by the private sector. At the global level, the increasing scope and power of large transnational corporations were reaching countries and populations across borders, ignoring or weakening the states' national sovereignty.

The new concept of 'governance', both at national and international levels, meant that states and intergovernmental organizations could no longer work on their own: they needed to ally themselves with other entities: civil society institutions, NGOs and, as an innovation, with the private commercial sector. In order to reduce global disparities in health, it was no longer sufficient to rely only on the public sector and on private voluntary efforts (NGOs, philanthropy) and to better coordinate traditional roles: the traditional approach had proved that it could not tackle and solve all the world's health problems. The new approach, for WHO and other health institutions, was therefore to enter into broad alliances and partnerships, to enlist the efforts of both the public and private sectors, in order to achieve a synergistic combination of the strengths, resources and expertise of all partners.

Initiatives, alliances and partnerships

Examples of the main initiatives, alliances and partnerships in which WHO has been involved are given hereunder, set in three groups.

Most of these initiatives, alliances and partnerships were formed to fight specific diseases or disease-producing addictions: see Presentation 11.1.

Presentation 11.1

**Public Health Initiatives,
Alliances and Partnerships to Fight Specific Diseases
or Disease-Producing Addictions**

- 1974: the Onchocerciasis Control Programme (OCP): WHO, World Bank, UNDP, FAO, governments – it has benefited from the free donation by Merck & Co. Mectizan® since 1989;
- 1988: the Global Polio Eradication Initiative: WHO, UNICEF, European Commission, governments, foundations, NGOs – largely promoted and supported by Rotary International, it has Aventis Pasteur as a corporate partner;
- 1996: the UN Programme on HIV/AIDS (UNAIDS): WHO, UNICEF, UNDP, UNFPA, UNESCO, World Bank, ILO, governments, foundations, NGOs – business partners include Glaxo Wellcome, F. Hoffman-La Roche, Virco N.V., Bristol-Myers Squibb, Organon Teknika;
- 1998: Roll Back Malaria: WHO, UNICEF, UNDP, World Bank, governments, foundations, NGOs, private sector firms – since 2001, Novartis provides developing countries with Coartem, at cost, as treatment for drug resistant malaria;
- 1998: The Tobacco Free Initiative: against the tobacco industry;
- 1998: The Global Alliance to Eliminate Lymphatic Filariasis: WHO, UNICEF, World Bank, governments, development agencies, research institutions, NGOs – Binax, Inc., Merck & Co., GlaxoSmithKline;
- 1999: *Stop TB* Initiative: WHO, World Bank, US CDCs, NGOs – involving the private sector in care implementation;
- 1999: WHO European Partnership Project on Tobacco Dependence, open to public and private partners: includes Glaxo Wellcome, Novartis and Pharmacia & Upjohn (treatment products for tobacco dependence);
- 2002: International HIV Treatment Coalition (ITAC): WHO, UNAIDS, governments, foundations, NGOs, private sector;
- 2002: The Measles Initiative: American and other Red Cross Societies, WHO, PAHO, UNICEF, governments, NGOs – no initial business involvement.

Other initiatives and partnerships have focused on access to vaccines and research of new vaccines: see Presentation 11.2.

Presentation 11.2

**Initiatives, Alliances and Partnerships on Access
to Vaccines and Research on New Vaccines**

- 1990: The Children's Vaccine Initiative (CVI): WHO, UNICEF, UNDP, World Bank, research groups, a foundation and the vaccine industry;
- 1996: International AIDS Vaccine Initiative (IAVI): World Bank, governments, foundations, policy makers and industry leaders;
- 1998: The Children's Vaccine Program: WHO, UNICEF, UNDP, World Bank, CVI, the International Vaccine Institute;
- 1999: The Global Alliance for Vaccines and Immunization: WHO, UNICEF, World Bank, governments, public health institutions, foundations, NGOs and the vaccine industry;
- 2000: HIV Vaccine Initiative: WHO, UNAIDS (with their partners);
- 2000: Accelerating Access Initiative: WHO, UNAIDS, UNICEF, UNFPA and six pharmaceutical companies: Abbott Laboratories, Boeringher Ingelheim, Bristol-Myers Squibb, GlaxoSmithKline, Hoffman La Roche and Pfizer.

WHO has also been associated with the private sector for the development of new drugs: see Presentation 11.3.

Presentation 11.3

Initiatives, Alliances and Partnerships for the Development of New Drugs

- 1999: WHO/Japan/Japanese Pharmaceutical companies: research of candidate antimalarials;
- 1999: Medicines for Malaria Venture (A Swiss Foundation): WHO, governments, foundations and IFPMA, ExxonMobil Corporation;
- 2000: Global Alliance for TB Drug Development: WHO, governments, foundations, NGOs, pharmaceutical and biotechnology companies – in 2002, it licenced a new drug candidate from Chiron Corporation;
- 2001: WHO/GlaxoSmithKline: development of LAPDAP, a new treatment for malaria;
- 2003: Drugs for Neglected Diseases Initiative: MSF, Institut Pasteur, the Kenya Medical Research Institute, the Oswaldo Cruz Foundation, the Indian Council of Medical Research and the Malaysian Ministry of Health, WHO/TDR.

WHO's interests and expectations

For WHO, the purpose of public-private partnerships and alliances is to harness the health industry's power, influence, technology and other resources as a complement to its own programmes. Obtaining more funds, when national and international public funding of health programmes was becoming scarce, was one part of WHO's motivation, but not the only one. The main point was that it was time for WHO, as well as for the other UN organizations in their own fields, to recognize and acknowledge the role of the private sector in the public health area and to work with, and not against, the health industry.

More resources from the private sector should strengthen campaigns for the eradication or control of specific diseases. They should accelerate research and development of new or neglected drugs, of vaccines. They should facilitate universal access to essential drugs and health services.

WHO and other public agencies benefit from working in collaboration with the private sector in areas not covered by their mandates, and/or where these organizations lack capacity, expertise and experience, e.g. in product research and development, manufacturing, marketing and distribution. Partnerships appear to be most justified where traditional ways of working independently have a limited impact on a problem; the specific desired goals can be agreed by the potential partners; the long-term interests of each sector are fulfilled (i.e. that there are benefits for all parties); there is relevant complementary expertise in both sectors; and the contributions of expertise and resources are reasonably balanced.

WHO also expects that partnerships would encourage industry to abide by the health-for-all principles, public health policies, WHO resolutions and international guidelines. In specific programmes, WHO expects to be recognized as the directing authority on the basis of its global health expertise and experience.

However, there are areas, such as public health policy-making and regulatory approval, where the concept of partnership with the private sector is not appropriate: standard-setting for product safety, efficacy and quality cannot be shared with for-profit enterprises (Widdus, 2001). For instance, WHO's Tropical Diseases Programme (TDR) should properly work closely with industry to develop new drugs. But a WHO official said that the Organization's essential drugs department should be 'totally fire-walled off, because we, through the expert committee, have to finally decide, independently, is this a good drug or not – is it recommendable, is it safe?' (Yamey, 2002).

WHO also needs to exert caution in not favouring one particular enterprise, nor favouring a particular product (medicine or vaccine) unless justified by the quality and/or availability of the product.

The industry's interests

In the 1990s, industry came to recognize the potential benefits of alliances with the UN, and, in the health field, with WHO and UNICEF. A systematic dialogue with the UN organizations would allow the voice (and interests) of world business to be better heard and considered. Involvement with UN agencies and their committees would allow business to influence decision-making.

Association with the 'worthy and virtuous' UN bodies, global organizations dedicated to maintaining peace and security, promoting economic development, protecting human rights and fighting against disease, could only be a benefit for business corporations, through 'image transfer'.

Private sector industry and business are accountable to their shareholders to produce profit, while international organizations are accountable to their Member States, and indirectly to their populations. WHO's objective 'the attainment by all peoples of the highest possible level of health' is not related to nor dependent on a profit criterion.

For business, public-private partnerships are also a vehicle for penetrating emerging markets. As quoted by Buse and Walt (2002:53):

> As the president of the medical systems unit of Becton Dickinson & Co. has said of one GPPP [global public-private partnership]: 'Of course we want to help eradicate neonatal tetanus, but we also want to stimulate the use of non-reusable injection devices, and to build relationships with ministries of health that might buy other products from us as their economies develop'.

This raises the lasting question of the compatibility of the objectives of public institutions and those of for-profit enterprises.

Risks

WHO and other public health institutions take risks when entering into alliances or partnerships with the private sector.

The partners are not equal. The power of transnational corporations in national and international economies, the political support they receive from rich countries' governments, their ability and inclination to override national and international legislative and regulatory obstacles, to influence decision-making of intergovernmental bodies such as WTO, their financial resources, have no match in the UN organizations. The five largest multinationals have revenues more than double the combined gross domestic product of the poorest 100 countries (HAI, 2000).

UN organizations are weak: they are dependent politically and financially on their masters, their Member States, and particularly the rich countries. Their strength lies in their power of influence based on their values contained in such documents as the UN Charter, human rights treaties, the WHO Constitution, the ILO Conventions, other international conventions and declarations. They represent the needs and interests of all countries and populations, including those of the poor. Their strength also lies with their expertise, their capacity to mobilize and act, their integrity.

In the health field, the industry has used its power, its influence, to infiltrate international organizations, attempt to 'buy' specialists, and bend scientific studies or experts' views towards their views and interests. Within WHO or its expert committees, the overt or covert pressures from industry may cause staff or consultants to apply self censorship on issues that may hurt or affect the interests of industry.

Another risk is for WHO to be associated with an industry or business enterprise which does not respect agreed scientific or technical standards, or uses unethical methods in marketing, sales, or in influencing governments, international organizations, scientists, physicians or the general public, in their favour.

Leaving aside the tobacco industry, an enemy and not a potential associate, the image of a number of commercial enterprises in the health field has become tainted. WHO's experience with the baby food industry has shown the continuous opposition of the industry to international regulation, its flawed alternative proposals of weak self-monitored codes of conduct, its rejection of any independent international monitoring.

Pharmaceutical companies give financial incentives to doctors to favour their products, to push certain treatments, to ignore cheaper generic drugs. They try to influence scientific studies. For instance, as reported in the *Washington Post,* Pharmacia Corp. funded a study to show that a medicine called Celebrex worked better than cheaper alternatives such as Ibuprofen. The study collected 12 months of data, which suggested no Celebrex advantage. Then, the authors selectively published the first six months of results, which purported to show that Celebrex had fewer side effects: it caused US patients to spend $3 billion unnecesssarily (Mallaby, 2002). In May 2003, the *New York Times* revealed that Cutter Biological, a division of the German pharmaceutical company Bayer, had sold millions of dollars of blood-clotting medicine for hemophiliacs – medicine that carried a high risk of transmitting AIDS – to Asia and Latin America in the mid-1980s, while selling a new, safer product in the West. Bayer denied these allegations (Bogdanich and Koll, 2003). Widespread litigation has started in the USA, following successful fights against asbestos and tobacco, against big pharmaceutical companies, charging that they have hidden the dangers of medicines which have harmed thousands of patients.

In a recent, caricatural, but real example in a related field, an industry went so far as to blackmail WHO and FAO into amending scientific findings expected to affect its financial interests. The US Sugar Association wrote to WHO threatening to bring pressure to end US funding for WHO – $406 million – and FAO if a report was not withdrawn (James, 2003). The WHO/FAO joint report on *Diet, Nutrition and the Prevention of Chronic Diseases* refers to the contribution of nutrition – and especially the role of saturated fats, sugars and salt and excessive consumption – to the major chronic diseases, i.e. cardiovascular diseases, cancers, diabetes and obesity. The report had been prepared by a team of leading nutrition scientists. An element of the report recommends that added sugars be limited to less than 10 per cent of daily calorie intake. The industry wanted the limit to be kept at 25 per cent.

These considerations stress the need for WHO and other public health institutions to devise and implement safeguards, so that they may benefit from industry's participation, without encroaching upon the organizations' mandate, nor tainting their integrity.

Principles and safeguards

In January 2001, a secretariat document on 'Guidelines on interaction with commercial enterprises to achieve health outcome' was approved by the WHO

Executive Board. Further measures were announced by the Director-General to complement the guidelines (see Chapter 2).

Essentially, when joining forces with the private sector, WHO should ensure that their enterprises give allegiance to WHO's objectives and policies, accept its role as 'directing and coordinating authority' in international public health work, follow its technical guidance and accept its evaluations. The record of potential donor companies and companies which seek to work with WHO should be assessed in relation to UN human rights standards and ILO conventions and WHO's policies and guidelines.[1] The record of companies currently in partnership with WHO should be subject to the same type of assessment. Such assessments should preferably be undertaken by an independent external body including governments, the secretariat, NGOs and industry representatives, – or by an interagency UN body, or by a multinational firm specializing in social audit.

WHO should insist on complete transparency on contractual agreements with all commercial enterprises. An independent external body should monitor and evaluate regularly all private sector interactions with WHO. Beyond the scrutiny of proposed and existing partnerships by IGOs with the private sector, there is a need for an independent global regulatory and global health governance.

The selection of countries involved in partnerships should be based on set criteria linked to the needs of the populations.

Dr J.D. Quick, a senior WHO official, has recommended the following principles to apply in partnerships (Quick, 2001):

> First, the focus of the endeavour should be appropriate. Not all areas of public-private interaction are. For instance, normative functions such as setting regulatory standards for pharmaceutical products may use information and views from the private sector, but the regulatory decision-making process should be ring-fenced to remain independent, and not undertaken in partnership.
>
> Second, the nature of each partner's involvement should be subject to certain expectations and conditions. For example, a public-private partnership for research and development of a new product must have a firewall between the overall management of the project and the scientific evaluation of the results. The freedom to publish both positive and negative results is vital to the scientific integrity of such a partnership.
>
> Third, each partner must maintain full independence in policy matters and in areas of endeavour outside the focus of the partnership. For WHO this means, among other things, continuing to speak out and to take action on matters of public policy, even where WHO's views may differ from those of its partners.

Other useful suggestions to WHO came out of an International Seminar on 'Global Public-Private Partnerships for Health and Equity' held on 23–24 November 2001 in Rome (Italy).[2] Among them:

- WHO needs to set the priorities for agenda setting of partnerships building on its technical capacity and scientific knowledge;
- WHO needs to look at its own governance structures at the highest level in terms of strategic priority setting for partnerships. It needs to be accountable, transparent and democratic in its own decision-making processes in order to have a logical rather than an ad hoc approach to partnerships;

- WHO's Guidelines need to be reviewed and to be placed in a broader conceptual framework that extends beyond bilateral interactions;
- WHO needs to strengthen its capacity to negotiate and engage with the profit and civil society sectors, to be clear when partnerships are not appropriate and, in such cases, to be prepared to say 'no' to potential donors;
- WHO needs to be accountable to the people and listen more to the peoples' needs in particular to the South's concerns and to empower civil society as an equal member of partnerships.

Access to essential medicines

Alliance and partnerships have not facilitated universal access to essential drugs and health services. Pharmaceutical companies have resisted price reductions of their products, including antiretrovirals, favouring country by country agreements. Price reductions have been obtained mainly because of pressures by NGOs and public opinion. The industry has resisted the increased use of generic drugs, and the production and sale of generic drugs in developing countries.

WHO's opening to business has not solved the dilemma: what is the appropriate balance between the needs of the poor population to have access to essential medicines at accessible costs, and the legitimate protection of pharmaceutical patents.

Health activists submit that access to essential medicines is part of the 'right to health' as defined by the Universal Declaration of Human Rights (Art. 25), the International Covenant on Economic, Social and Cultural Rights (Art. 12), the Convention on the Right of the Child (Art. 24). It should therefore be considered as a fundamental human right. The Preamble of the WHO Constitution states that 'The enjoyment of the highest attainable standard of health is one of the fundamental rights of every human being without distinction of race, religion, political belief, economic or social condition'. It also states that 'Governments have a responsibility for the health of their peoples which can be fulfilled only by the provision of adequate health and social measures'.

These texts refer to the right to a 'standard of living adequate for the health ... including ... medical care', or the right to the 'highest attainable standard of physical and mental health', or the right of the child's 'access to ... health care services'. There is however no specific reference to a right to access to medical medicines at reasonable prices, even if such access is required in order to provide essential health services to poor and sick populations. Furthermore, the promotion and protection of human rights is a responsibility of governments.

At best, access to essential drugs at reasonable prices could be considered as a desirable, non-legally binding, human right.[3]

On the other hand, the protection of patents is legally enforceable at the national level. The patent system has been strengthened in 1994 by the incorporation of a regime for protecting intellectual property rights, the TRIPS Agreements. Failure to respect TRIPS may expose a state to WTO complaints and subsequent sanctions. A transition period has been granted to developing countries, but total compliance with patent protection will then be required. Some exceptions are allowed, such as compulsory licences, under certain conditions. Such conditions may be waived in times of national emergencies, such as HIV/AIDS crises in Africa (see Chapter 4).

Pharmaceutical companies have been criticized for charging high prices for drugs sold in developing countries, particularly antiretrovirals. They reply that high prices are necessary in order to provide innovation in the pharmaceutical field: lowering prices might limit R&D, and the production of new, more effective medicines. While this argument is generally dismissed as not valid and an empty threat, the industry then retreats to the better argument that healthcare is the responsibility of governments, not of business firms. Klaus Schwab, president and founder of the World Economic Forum, has deplored that the responsibility for fighting poverty, guaranteeing public health and protecting the environment has been handed over to corporations 'as if businesses were bottomless pits of money whose sole function was to provide social benefits to the world'. He believe that this trend has gone too far: 'After all, economic growth is the business of business' (Schwab, 2003).

If the business of business is business, WHO's business is global public health: the organization cannot be neutral with regard to the access of essential medicines to poor populations. The World Health Assembly has requested the secretariat to 'pursue all diplomatic and political opportunities aimed at overcoming barriers to access to essential medicines'. WHO should therefore continue its efforts to inform countries about the public health implications of the TRIPS Agreements for access to essential medicines. As recommended in Chapter 2 (Conclusion), WHO should take a more activist role in supporting a 'health exception' in WTO debates and negotiations. It should advocate that differential pricing become more systematic, as recommended by MSF, HAI and Oxfam at the World Health Assembly in May 2003 (MSF, 2003c). It should continue to promote generic drugs.

At the same time, WHO has to maintain a reasonable degree of collaboration with the pharmaceutical industry in its various alliances and partnerships, particularly in view of the industry's unique and essential role in R&D for neglected drugs and for vaccines. An open conflict 'against' the pharmaceutical industry would probably be counter-productive for WHO, and therefore for public health: it should be avoided.

In the final analysis, the onus is with governments: the role of the WHO secretariat is to influence governments, with the support of like-minded countries and NGOs, in order to facilitate and develop the access of all populations to essential medicines at reasonable prices.

Conclusion

According to Health Action International (HAI, 2000), the most important question is whether increased interaction with the commercial sector is a major way forward towards Health for All. WHO must be able to demonstrate that the poor directly benefit from such interaction, and from more public-private alliances and partnerships.

No such demonstration has yet been made. The resistance opposed by the pharmaceutical industry to reduce the prices of medicines for developing countries, thus limiting the access of poor populations to effective treatment, shows that WHO cannot relinquish its obligations to protect and enhance the health of poor populations.

On the other hand, the list of Initiatives, Alliances and Partnerships given in Presentations 11.1, 11.2 and 11.3 shows that a number of specific health partnerships with the private sector is playing a useful role as a complement to the contributions of the UN organizations, NGOs and foundations, or in some areas, a necessary role.

For instance, the open-ended donation by Merck & Co. to the onchocerciasis programme; the participation of Aventis Pasteur to the Global Polio Eradication Initiative, although Rotary International is here the main external supporter of the programme; the use of Novartis' Coartem in the Malaria programme; the participation of several pharmaceutical companies in the Lymphatic Filariasis Alliance and in the fight against TB.

Both public and private institutions, and particularly the major pharmaceutical companies, play a necessary role in research and development of prevention and treatment medicines to combat HIV/AIDS, malaria and TB. Their participation is again essential for R&D for new vaccines and to engage in R&D of drugs for neglected diseases.

While public-private partnerships for health are here to stay, the increased number of partnerships associating WHO with the private, for-profit, sector requires that independent research be carried out on the risks and benefits of such ventures, on desirable guidelines (should the present Guidelines be tightened?), and on how WHO has managed, so far, this innovation. Independent assessments should also be made on each of the past and current partnerships, and decisions made about the continuation or the cessation of current partnerships.

In the words of Quick (2001), public-private partnerships can harness private expertise, creativity, and resources for the public good. Much can be achieved through well-conceived and effectively implemented partnerships.

However, a principled approach is needed to ensure that the focus of the partnership is appropriate, that the involvement of each partner is subject to certain expectations and conditions, and that each partner maintains independence in policy matters and endeavours outside the partnership.

At the same time, one agrees with Widdus (2001): public-private partnerships are social experiments that are attempting to learn how to tackle intractable health problems in better ways. Partnerships can be helpful but are not a panacea. They are one of many different approaches to combat disease and promote public health on a global basis.

The interaction between public health institutions and for-profit enterprises needs close oversight and better regulation. In its interaction with the private sector, WHO must retain its own identity, implement its international public health mandate and protect its integrity.

Notes

1   A first step has been taken with the approval on 13 August 2003 by the UN Commission for the Promotion and Protection of Human Rights of the Draft Norms on the

Responsibilities of Transnational Corporations and Other Business Enterprises with Regard to Human Rights'. The Norms would still need to be adopted by governments or companies, then monitoring by independent bodies should follow.
2   The Seminar was organized by the Society for International Development, WHO and the Istituto Superiore di Sanita.
3   For a more detailed discussion of this issue, see Sarah Joseph, 'Pharmaceutical Corporations and Access to Drugs: the Fourth Wave of Corporate Human Rights Scrutiny', in *Human Rights Quarterly,* Vol. 25, No. 2, 2003, pp. 425–452.

Bibliography

Ahya (2002), 'Islam's Solution to Aids', Ahya.org, English Resources.

Allain, A. (Ed.)(1986), *Milk and Murder, Address by Dr. Cecily Williams to the Rotary Club of Singapore in 1939*, Penang: International Organization of Consumers Unions (IOCU).

Anello, E. (2001), 'Consultant Report, Assessing Conflict of Interest', WHO (unpublished) report, 21 June.

Armada, F., Muntaner, C. and Navarro, V.(2001), 'Health and Social Security Reforms in Latin America: The Convergence of the World Health Organization, the World Bank, and Transnational Corporations', *International Journal of Health Services*, Vol. 31, No. 4, pp. 729–768.

Armstrong, H. (1999), 'UNICEF: Lessons Learned from the Baby-Friendly Hospital Initiative', *Women Friendly Health Services – Experience in Maternal Care: A Report of a WHO/UNICEF/UNFPA Workshop, Mexico City, January 26–28, 1999*, UNICEF.

Ashraf, H., (2001), 'WHO Commission announces bold plan for world's poor', *The Lancet*, Vol. 358, 22/29 December, p. 2133.

Aventis (undated), Aventis Pasteur, Community involvement, 'GAVI Partnerships'.

Backus, D. and Cabral, L. (2001), 'Merck, AIDS and Africa', Firms and Markets, Mini-Case, NYU Stern, 31 August.

Baker, R. (2003), 'Bush Plan for $15 Billion to Combat AIDS in Africa Stuns Friends and Foes Alike', HIV and AIDS Top Stories, 28 January 2003.

Bale Jr, H. (2002), 'WHO: the casualties and compromises of renewal', letter in *The Lancet*, Vol. 360, 21 September, p. 953–954.

Baue, W. (2002), 'Rio + 10 Series: UNAIDS Accelerating Access Initiative May Decelerate Access', 19 July.

BBC (2001a), 'Glaxo offers cheaper AIDS drugs', BBC News Business, 21 February.

BBC (2001b), 'US drops Brazil AIDS drugs case', BBC News Business, 25 June.

Becker, E. (2002), 'Trade talks on low-cost drugs fail', International Herald Tribune, 23 December.

Beigbeder, Y. (1997), 'Another role for an NGO: financing a WHO programme, Rotary International and the Eradication of Poliomyelitis', *Transnational Associations*, January, pp. 37–43.

Beigbeder, Y. (1998), with the collaboration of M. Nashat, M.-A. Orsini and J.-F. Tiercy, *The World Health Organization*, Martinus Nijhoff Publishers, The Hague/London/Boston.

Beigbeder, Y. (2001), *New Challenges for UNICEF, Children, Women and Human Rights*, Palgrave, Basingstoke.

Bellamy, C. (1999), Letter from Carol Bellamy, Executive Director of UNICEF, to Peter Brabeck-Letmathe, Chief Executive Officer, Nestlé SA, 31 December.

Bello, W. (2002), 'Learning from Doha: A Civil Society Perspective from the South', *Global Governance*, Vol. 8, No. 3, July-September, pp. 273–279.

Benkimoun, P. (2003), 'L'UE veut relancer les négociations sur l'accès aux médicaments', *Le Monde*, 11 January.

Birmingham, M.E. *et al*, (1996?) 'Overview of the Global Polio Eradication Initiative', internal unpublished WHO document.

Black, M. (1996), *Children First, The Story of UNICEF, Past and Present*, UNICEF, Oxford University Press, Oxford/New York.

Blanks, J. et al (1998), 'The Onchocerciasis Elimination Program for the Americas: a historical partnership', *Rev Panam Salud Publica*, 3 June (6): 367–74.

Bodenheimer, T. (2000), 'Uneasy Alliance, Clinical Investigators and the Pharmaceutical Industry', *The New England Journal of Medicine*, Vol. 342, No. 20, 18 May, pp. 1539–1543.

Bogdanich, W. and Koll, E. (2003), 'Bayer sold drug in Third World despite AIDS taint', *International Herald Tribune*, 25 May.

Bruno, K. and Karliner, J. (2000), 'Tangled Up in Blue, Corporate Partnerships at the United Nations', 1 September. www.corpwatch.org/campaigns/PCD.jsp?articleid=996

Buse, K. and Walt, G. (2002), 'Globalization and multilateral public-private health partnerships: issues for health policy', in K. Lee, K. Buse and S. Fustukian (eds), *Health Policy in a Globalising World*, Cambridge University Press, Cambridge, pp. 41–62.

CBS (2003), 'Drug Firm To Help Break AIDS Logjam', CBSNEWS.com, *Health*, 27 January.

Charatan, F. (2001), 'News, Bayer cuts price of ciprofloxacin after Bush threatens to buy generics', *British Medical Journal*, vol 323, 3 November.

Chetley, A. (1986), 'Health Action International, A profile of the action network that holds the pharmaceutical industry accountable', *New Internationalist*, Issue 165, November.

Collin, J., Lee, K. & Bissell, K. (2002), 'The framework convention on tobacco control: the politics of global health governance', *Third World Quarterly*, Vol. 23, No. 2, pp. 265–282.

CorpWatch (2001a), 'UN and Corporations Fact Sheet', 22 March 2001, www.corpwatch.org/campaigns/PCD.jcp?articleid=614

CorpWatch (2001b), 'The Meaning of Doha', W. Bello and A. Mittal, *Focus on the Global South and Food First*, 15 November.

De Young, K. (2001), 'The Catholic Church: AIDS, Condoms and the Roman Catholic Church', *The Washington Post*, 13 August.

Dunne, J. (2002), 'A word in anguish', *Drugs Quarterly*, 6(1): 2.

Dyer, O. (2002), 'Unicef comes under attack for Big Mac funding deal', *British Medical Journal*, vol. 325, 26 October.

Economist, The (2002a), 'Special report Aids in Southern Africa, Fighting back', 11 May.

Economist, The (2002b), 'South Africa and AIDS, Stop denying the killer bug', 23 February.

Feachem, R., Medlin, C., Daniels, D., Mshinda, H., Petko, J. *et al* (2002), 'Achieving impact: Roll Back Malaria in the next phase', Final Report of the external evaluation of Roll Back Malaria, 20 August, http://mosquito.who.int/ cmc_upload/0/000/015/905/ee.pdf

Ferriman, A. (2000), 'News, WHO accused of stifling debate about infant feeding', and Letters, *BMJ*, 320 (7246):1362 – 321 (7266): 956, 960, 20 May.

GAVI (2002a), 'The International Federation of Pharmaceutical Manufacturers Associations (IFPMA)', 5 February.

GAVI (2002b), '10.5 Million Children Vaccinated Against Hepatitis B', *Press Release*, 20 November.

GAVI (2003), 'GAVI and The Vaccine Fund Announce $60 Million Boost to Accelerate Development of Life-saving Vaccines', *Press Release*, 11 February.

Gellene, D. (2002), 'AIDS drug failure shakes VaxGen', *International Herald Tribune*, 28 February.

Gilmartin, R. (2002), 'Towards a healthy world, Health, trade and development', *OECD Observer Supplement*, Forum 2002, 15 May.

Global (2002), 'UK Working Group Report Provides Necessary Framework To Increase Access To Essential Medicines In The Developing World', Global Business Coalition on HIV/AIDS, 28 November.

Global Fund (2002), 'Global Fund to fight AIDS, tuberculosis and malaria announces first grants', Global Fund *Press Release*, 19 May.

Go Between (2002), 'Global Compact & GRI Cooperative Framework', No. 91, April–May.

Grunwald, M. (2002), 'Guns blaze in Bostwana war on AIDS, but old ways persist', *International Herald Tribune*, 3 December.

HAI (2000), 'Public-Private "Partnerships", Addressing Public Health Needs or Corporate Agendas', Introduction by Lisa Hayes, HAI Europe, 3 November.

HAI (2001), 'Public interest NGOs demand that the Global Health Fund meets poor countries' needs, not those of industry', HAI *Press Release,* 14 May.

HAI (2002), 'Statement for the WHO Executive Board, 14–21 January by Consumers International (CI), Health Action International (HAI), Médecins Sans Frontières (MSF), OXFAM delivered by Ellen't Hoen on 15 January' to the 109th Session of the WHO Executive Board, www.haiweb.org/campaign/access/ EB109statement.html

Hamm, B. (2002) 'The Global Compact, A Forum for Dialogue between the UN and Private Business', *D+C*, 4/02, pp. 20–26.

Hardon, A. (2001), 'Immunization for All ?, A crirical look at the first GAVI partners meeting', *HAI-Lights*, HAI Europe, Vol.6, No.1, March.

Herbert, B. (2001), 'A Lesson from Economics 101 at Big Tobacco University', *International Herald Tribune,* 24 July.

IARC (1986), 'Monograph on Tobacco Smoking', Vol. 38.

IARC (2002), 'Monograph on Tobacco Smoking and Smoke', Vol. 83.

IAVI (2003), 'AIDS Vaccine Trial Begins in Entebbe, Uganda', IAVI, 10 February.

IBFAN (1998), 'Breaking the Rules, Stretching the Rules, A Worldwide Report on Violations of the WHO/UNICEF International Code of Marketing of Breast-milk Substitutes', IBFAN, Penang.

IBFAN (2000), 'Does Nestlé's Monitoring Report Comply with the International Code ?', IBFAN News, April.

IBFAN (2001a), 'Breaking the Rules 2001', www.ibfan.org/english

IBFAN (2001b), 'The Issue, History of the Campaign', www.ibfan.org/english/issue/history01.html

IBFAN (2002), 'The optimal duration of exclusive breastfeeding', Breastfeeding Briefs No. 31 and 32.

Infact (2002), 'Japan Tobacco Documents Reveal Concerted Campaign Against Tobacco Treaty', 23 January.

Infact (2003), 'Treaty Trespassers: New Evidence of Escalating Tobacco Industry Activity to Derail the Framework Convention on Tobacco Control', February.

James, B. (2003), 'Sugar interests hit at UN study on illness links', *International Herald Tribune*, 23 April.

Joint Inspection Unit (JIU,1999), *Private Sector Involvement and Cooperation with the United Nations System*, Mezzalama, F., Ouedraogo, L.D., UN Doc. JIU/REP/99/6, Geneva.

Joint Inspection Unit (JIU, 2002), *Involvement of Civil Society Organizations other than NGOs and the Private Sector in Technical Cooperation Activities: Experiences and Prospects of the United Nations System*, Mezzalama, F., UN Doc. JIU/REP/2002/1, Geneva, February, p. 3.

Jones, P.M. (2001) 'Brazil's free AIDS-drug program slashes cases, earns global interest', *Media-AIDS*, 2 January.

JOURN-AIDS (2002), 'Africa: International coalition on antiretrovirals launched', 13 December.

Kapp, C. (2001a), 'WHO demands tighter voluntary tobacco controls', *The Lancet*, Vol. 358, 10 November.

Kapp, C. (2001b), 'More differences emerge at WHO tobacco talks', *The Lancet*, Vol. 357, 5 May.

Koivusalo, M. and Ollila, E. (1997), *Making a Healthy World, Agencies, Actors and Policies in International Health*, Stakes, Helsinki, Zed Books Ltd, London and New York.

Lamy, P. (2003), 'Access to medicines, Show the world that we can act', *International Herald Tribune*, 11–12 January.

Lancet, The (2001), 'The tightening grip of big pharma', Vol. 357, p. 1141, 14 April.

Langley, A. (2003a), 'US to back tobacco-control treaty, Despite earlier opposition, officials will not seek changes', *International Herald Tribune*, 19 May.

Langley, A. (2003b), 'WHO tobacco pact faces opposition', *International Herald Tribune*, 3 March.

Leisenger, K. M. (2002), 'The pharmaceutical industry and social responsibility: idealism without illusion and realism without resignation', Lecture at Berlin, 1 October, www.novartisfoundation.com

Mallaby, S. (2002), 'A worm of corruption at capitalism's core', *International Herald Tribune*, 11 June.

McManus, J., and Saywell, T., (2002), 'New Cures for An Old Killer', *Far Eastern Economic Review*, 7 March, pp. 26–28.

McNeil, D.G. (2001), 'Indian Company Offers to Supply AIDS Drugs at Low Cost in Africa', *The New York Times*, 7 February.

Merck (2003), 'Merck announces Fourth-Quarter 2002 Earnings Per Share (EPS) of 83 Cents, Full-Year 2002 EPS of $3.14', *Financial News*.

MSF (2001), 'Pretoria, Joint MSF-Oxfam-Treatment Action Campaign Press Release', 19 April, www.accessmed-msf.org/ms

MSF (2002a), 'G8: Drugs for neglected diseases', J. Orbinski and B. Pecoul, 21 June, www.accessmed-msf./org/ms

MSF (2002b), 'WHO's essential drugs list should go hand in hand with prices', www.msf.org/co.../page.cfm?articleid=01607 9 February.

MSF (2002c), 'What is the cost and who will pay', *MSF Report* on "Changing national malaria treatment protocols in Africa", 13 February.

MSF (2003a), 'No consensus at the TRIPS Council but a last opportunity to fix flaws in the TRIPS Agreement', 7 January.

MSF (2003b), 'G8: Unkept promises', MSF Website, May.

MSF (2003c), 'MSF, Oxfam, HAI Note to WHO member country delegations at the 56th World Health Assembly', 13 May.

Nabarro, D.N. and Tayler, E.M. (1998), 'The "Roll Back Malaria" Campaign', *Science*, Vol. 280, 26 June, pp. 2067–2068.

Nakajima, H. (1995), 'WHO chief blames tobacco industry greed for killer "pandemic"', *U.N. Observer and International Report*, July 1995, p.5.

Nelson, J. (2002), *Building Partnerships, Cooperation between the United Nations system and the private sector*, Report commissioned by the UN Global Compact Office, UN/DPI-The Prince of Wales International Business Leaders Forum, p.2.

Newsweek (2003), 'The Last Word Dr Lee Jong-wook, Impress Girls: Saves Lives', Interview with A.A. Seno, 28 July.

Normile, D. (2003), 'Novartis Kick Off Institute for Neglected Diseases', *Science*, Vol. 299, 7 February.

Nullis, C. (2003), 'Health Activists Slam New Draft Tobacco Treaty as Feeble', *Associated Press*, 15 January.

Ong, E.K., Glantz, S.A.(2000), 'Tobacco industry efforts subverting International Agency for Research on Cancer' second-hand smoke study', *The Lancet*, Vol. 355: 1253–59, 8 April.

Oxfam (2002a), 'TRIPS and Public Health, The next battle', Oxfam Briefing Paper, 15 March.

Oxfam (2002b), 'Oxfam condemns deadlock on access to affordable medicines negotiations', Press Release, 21 December.

Oxfam (2002c), 'Generic competition, price and access to medicines, The case of anti-retrovirals in Uganda', Oxfam Briefing Paper, 10 July.

Oxfam (2002d), 'Global Fund in danger of delivering little more than false hope, says Oxfam International', *Oxfam International Press Release*, 5 July.

Palmedo, M. (2002), 'Chiron & TB Alliance licensing deal for pipeline TB drug', http://www.tballiance.org/popup_chiron.cfm?rm=press, 13 February.

Paulson, T. (2001), 'GAVI's goal is clear, even if route to it is not', *Seattle Post-Intelligencer*, 23 March.

Pear, R. and Oppel Jr, R.A. (2002), 'Drug industry seeks profit from US electoral victories', *International Herald Tribune*, 22 November.

Quick, J.D. (2001), 'Partnerships need principles', *Bulletin of the World Health Organization*, 79 (8), p. 776.

Rabe, H.-J. (2002), 'Public Private Partnerships, A Model with a future in Development Cooperation', *D+C*, 4/02, pp. 9–11.

Ramsay, S. (2002), 'Global Fund makes historic first round of payments', *The Lancet*, Vol. 359, 4 May 2002, pp. 1581–1582.

Richards, F.O. Jr. *et al.* (2002), 'The Carter Center's assistance to river blindness control programs: establishing treatment objectives and goals for monitoring ivermectin delivery systems on two continents', *American Journal of Tropical Medicine and Hygiene*, Aug;65(2): 108–14.

Richter, J. (2001), *Holding Corporations Accountable: Corporate Conduct, International Codes and Citizen Action*, UNICEF, Zed Books, London/New York.

Roll Back Malaria (2002), RBM Infosheet, WHO, March.

Rosenthal, E. (2002), 'China acknowledges it has an AIDS epidemic and asks for help', *International Herald Tribune*, 7–8 September.

Ruggie, J.G. (2000), 'Globalization, the Global Compact and corporate social responsibility', *Transnational Associations*, 6/2000, pp. 291–294.

Ruggie, J.G. (2001), 'The Global Compact as Learning Network', *Global Governance*, Vol. 7, No. 4 Oct.-Dec. pp. 371–378.

Save the Children UK (2002), 'A Long Way to Go: a critique of GAVI's initial impact', *Briefing analysis*, January, revised March.

Schwab, K. (2003), 'Get Back to Business', *Newsweek*, 5 May.

Shubber, S. (1985), 'The International Code of Marketing of Breast-milk Substitutes', *International Digest of Health Legislation*, Vol. 36, No. 4, pp. 877–908.

Shubber, S. (1998), *The International Code of Marketing of Breast-milk Substitutes: An International Measure to Protect and Promote Breast-feeding*, Kluwer Law International, The Hague/London/Boston.

Swarns, R. (2002), 'South Africa to offer AIDS drugs', *International Herald Tribune*, 19 April.

Taylor, A. (1998), 'Monitoring the international code of marketing of breast-milk substitutes: an epidemiological study in four countries', *British Medical Journal*, Vol. 316, pp. 117–22.

Tecklehaimanot, A., Snow, R.W. (2002), 'Will the Global Fund help roll back malaria in Africa?', *The Lancet*, Vol. 360, 21 September.

Tesner, S. (2000), *The United Nations and Business, A Partnership Recovered*, Macmillan, Basingstoke.

Thomas, C. (2002), 'Trade policy and the politics of access to drugs', *Third World Quarterly*, Vol. 23, No. 2, pp.251–264.

UN (2001), 'Declaration of Commitment on HIV/AIDS, Global Crisis – Global Action', Doc. A/s-26/L.2, 27 June.

UN Foundation (2002), 'New Tobacco Control Text Planned for WHO Meeting', *UN Wire*, 11 October.

UNAIDS (2000a), 'Preventing Mother-to-Child HIV Transmission: Technical Experts Recommend Use of Antiretroviral Regimens Beyond Pilot Projects', UNAIDS *Press Release*, 25 October.

UNAIDS (2000b), 'New public/private sector effort initiated to accelerate access to HIV/AIDS care and treatment in developing countries', UNAIDS *Press Release*, 11 May.

UNAIDS (2001), 'Top Businesses Pledge to Act on HIV/AIDS', UNAIDS *Press Release*, 26 June.

UNAIDS (2002a), 'New UNAIDS report warns AIDS epidemic still in early phase and not leveling off in worst affected countries', UNAIDS *Press Release*, 2 July.

UNAIDS (2002b), 'Report on the Global HIV/AIDS Epidemic 2002', UNAIDS, July.

UNAIDS (2002c), 'Initiative to promote access to quality HIV medicines releases first batch of rresults today', Joint UNAIDS/UNICEF/WHO *Press Release*, 20 March.

UNAIDS/WHO (2001), 'Secretary-General advances plans for international AIDS and health fund', UNAIDS/WHO *Press Release* WHA54/4, 17 May.

UNICEF (1993), 'Facts for Life'.

UNICEF (1999a), 'Statement of UNICEF Executive Director Carol Bellamy to Harvard International Development, Conference on "Sharing responsibilities: public, private and civil society"', 19 April.

UNICEF (1999b), 'Breastfeeding: foundation for a healthy future'.

UNICEF (2001), 'Africa Receives First Delivery of GAVI/Global Fund Vaccines', *Press Release*, 6 April.

UNICEF (2002a), 'Five leading global health organizations anounce initiative to save children from measles deaths as part of a global effort to reduce child mortality', *Press Release*, 6 February.

UNICEF (2002b), 'Business-like approach to funding health programs in poor countries may save more than two million lives in 5 years', *Press Centre*, 1 February.

United Nations (1998), *Report of the Secretary-General on the Work of the Organization – 1998*, UN Doc. A/53/1, Introduction, paras. 10, 11.

United Nations (2002), *The Global Compact: Report on Progress and Activities*, Global Compact Office, July.

United Nations Association of the United States of America (2000), 'Business, the UN and the millennium: Where are we?', *The InterDependent*, Vol. 25, No. 4, p. 12, Winter.

US (2000), 'Surgeon General Satcher Says US Committed To Strong Global Treaty To Curb Tobacco', US Mission Geneva *Press Release*, 12 October.

US (2002a), 'USTR Explains Proposal for Health Emergency Drug Licensing', US Mission Geneva *Daily Bulletin*, 25 June.

US (2002b), 'US Releases Special 301 Report on Intellectual Property', US Department of State, International Information Programs, 30 April.

Utting, P. (2001), 'UN-business partnerships: whose agenda counts?', *Transnational Associations*, pp. 118–129.

Weiss, T.G. and Gordenker, L. (Eds)(1996), *NGOs, the UN, and Global Governance*, Lynne Rienner, Boulder, London.

WHO (1981), *International Code of Marketing of Breast-milk Substitutes*, WHO.

WHO (1987), 'Behaviour of nongovernmental organizations (NGOs) during Health Assemblies', WHO Doc. EB81/NGO/WP/1, 4 December, p. 24.

WHO (1988), *Guidelines on National Drug Policies*, Geneva: WHO.

WHO (1990), 'Review of nongovernmental organizations in official relations with WHO', WHO Doc. EB85/36, 22 January 1990, para. 13.

WHO (1996a), *The Reform of the World Bank and its Implications for Health Development*, WHO/INA/96.2.

WHO (1996b), 'The tobacco epidemic: a global public health emergency', *Fact Sheet* No. 118, May.

WHO (1997a), 'Polio, The beginning of the end', WHO, Geneva, 1997, pp. 5–6.

WHO (1997b), 'Tobacco epidemic: health dimensions', *Fact Sheet* No. 154, May.

WHO (1997c), 'Tobacco epidemic: much more than a health issue', *Fact Sheet* No. 155, May.

WHO (1997d), 'Governments for a tobacco-free world', *Fact Sheet* No. 159, May.

WHO (1997e), 'Tobacco epidemic in the Western Pacific', *Fact Sheet* No. 175, August.

WHO (1997f), 'United for a tobacco-free world', *Press Release* WHO/42, 28 May.

WHO (1998a), *Dr Gro Harlem Brundtland, Director-General Elect, Speech to the Fifty-first World Health Assembly, Geneva, 13 May 1998*, WHO Doc. A/51/DIV/6, 13 May.

WHO (1998b), *Director-General implements new code of conduct for financial disclosure*, Press Release WHO/55, 21 July.

WHO (1998c), 'Four International Organizations unite to roll back malaria', *Press Release* WHO/77, 30 October.

WHO (1998d), 'Dr Gro Harlem Brundtland elected Director-General of the World Health Organization', *Press Release* WHA/3, 13 May.

WHO (1999a), 'WHO in Partnership: Examples of Work with the Public and Private Sectors to Fight Infectious Diseases', WHO *Fact Sheet* No. 235, October.

WHO (1999b), 'Public-private partnerships for health, Report by the Director-General', WHO Doc. EB105/8, 14 December.

WHO (1999c), 'Backgrounder, Trade and Public Health, Why the World Health Organization is at the Third Ministerial Conference of the World Trade Organization', Seattle, 30 November to 3 December.

WHO (1999d), 'WHO calls for good drug donation practice during emergencies as it issues new *Guidelines*', *Press Release* WHO/45, 3 September 1999, and Doc. WHO/EDM/PAR/99.4, 'Guidelines for Drug Donation'.

WHO (1999e), 'New Partners join major offensive to rid the world of polio in 18 months', *Press Release* WHO/38, 7 July.

WHO (1999f), 'Poliomyelitis', *Press Release,* 7 December.

WHO (1999g), 'WHO, partner agencies and industry launch unique venture to develop malaria drugs', *Press Release* WHO/IFPMA, 3 November.

WHO (1999h), 'Japanese Government, pharmaceutical companies to join WHO in effort to find more effective anti-malarial drugs', *Press Release* WHO/63, 26 October.

WHO (1999i), 'WHO launches partnership with the pharmaceutical industry to help smokers quit', *Press Release* WHO/4, 30 January.

WHO (1999j), 'Cigarettes should be regulated like other drugs, says Director-General', *Press Release* WHO/26, 26 April.

WHO (1999k), 'Nowhere to run – nowhere to hide, WHO launches ground-breaking global campaign to counter tobacco industry deception', *Press Release* WHO, 4 November.

WHO (2000a), 'Tobacco company strategies to undermine tobacco control activities at the World Health Organization: report of the Committee of Experts on Tobacco Industry Documents'.

WHO (2000b), 'Onchocerciasis (River Blindness)', *Fact Sheet* No. 95, Rev. February.

WHO (2000c), 'Public-private partnerships for health, Medicines for Malaria Venture', Doc. EB105/8 Add.1, 6 January.

WHO (2000d), 'Children's Immunization Campaign Launched at World Economic Forum, Gates Foundation money to spur fight against preventable diseases', *Press Release* WHO/GAVI, 31 January.

WHO (2001a) Doc. EB107/2001/REC/2, 19 January, pp. 156, 159.

WHO (2001b), Legal Counsel's statement in Doc. EB107/SR/12, 22 January, p. 6.

WHO (2001c), *Declaration of Interests,* (internal) Cluster Note 2001/27, 21 September.

WHO (2001d), 'Public-private interactions for health: WHO's involvement, Note by the Director-General', Doc. EB109/4, 5 December.

WHO (2001e), 'Childhood nutrition and progress in implementing the International Code of Marketing of Breast-milk Substitutes, Report by the Secretariat', Doc. EB109/11, 11 December, paragraph 19.

WHO (2001f), 'WHO medicines strategy, Expanding access to essential drugs, Report by the Secretariat', Doc. EB109/7, 11 December.

WHO (2001g), 'WHO medicines strategy, Revised procedure for updating WHO's Model List of Essential Drugs, Report by the Secretariat', Doc. EB109/8, 7 December.

WHO (2001h), 'WHO/WTO Workshop on Pricing and Financing of Essential Drugs, Experts: Affordable Medicines for Poor Countries are Feasible', *Press Release* WHO/20, 11 April.

WHO (2001i), 'Statement by the WHO on the outcome of the WTO's Doha Ministerial Conference 2001', Statement WHO/18, 15 November.

WHO (2001j), 'Affordable AIDS drugs are within reach', *Note for the Press No.2,* 14 February.

WHO (2001k), 'Poliomyelitis', *Fact Sheet* No. 114, Rev. April.

WHO (2001l), 'GlaxoSmithKline and WHO sign agreement to develop a new treatment for malaria', *Press Release* WHO/10, 2 March.

WHO (2001m), 'WHO and Novartis join forces to combat drug resistant malaria', *Press Release,* WHO/26, 23 May.

WHO (2001n), 'WHO framework convention on tobacco control, Report by the Secretariat', Doc. A54/13, 2 April.

WHO (2002a), WHO Doc. EB109/SR2, 14 January, p. 14.

WHO (2002b), 'WHO Report outlines plan for new health spending – points to way out of poverty', *Press Release* WHO/06, 31 January.

WHO (2002c), 'Childhood nutrition and progress in implementing the International Code of Marketing of Breast-milk Substitutes, Report by the Secretariat', Doc. A55/14, 19 March.

WHO (2002d), 'Infant and young child nutrition, Global Strategy on infant and young child feeding, Report by the Secretariat', Doc. A/55/15, 16 April.

WHO (2002e), 'Essential Drugs and Medicines Policy – The Rationale of Essential Drugs, – Access Strategy, – Financing Mechanisms', www.who.int/edm.

WHO (2002f), Doc. EB109/SR/4, 15 January, pp. 3 and 4.

WHO (2002g), '3 million HIV/AIDS sufferers could receive antiretroviral therapy by 2005', *Press Release* WHO/58, 9 July.

WHO (2002h), 'Poliomyelitis', *Fact Sheet* No. 114, Rev. August.

WHO (2002i), 'West Africa launches final assault on polio – 60 million children to be vaccinated', *Press Release*, 12 November.

WHO (2002j), 'Tuberculosis', *Fact Sheet* No. 104, Revised August.

WHO (2002k), 'Low investment in immunization and vaccines threatens Global Health', *Press Release*, 20 November.

WHO (2002l), 'Low investment in immunization and vaccines threatens Global Health', *Press Release*, 20 November.

WHO (2003a), 'WHO Director-General calls India "number 1" polio era priority', *Press Release*, 7 April.

WHO (2003b), 'Malaria is alive and well and killing more than 3000 African children every day, WHO and UNICEF call for urgent increased efforts to roll back malaria', *Press Release* WHO/33, 25 April.

WHO (2003c), 'WHO reports 10 million TB patients successfully treated under "DOTS" 10 years after declaring TB a Global Emergency', *Press Release*.

WHO (2003d), 'Health Impact', Tobacco Free Initiative (undated), accessed 13 July.

WHO (2003e), 'New WHO Director-General urges countries to sign Tobacco Convention', *Press Release* WHO/62, 4 August.

WHO Bulletin (2001), 'TB drugs slashed for poor countries', 79(9), p. 904.

WHO/UNAIDS (2000), 'WHO and UNAIDS join forces to launch HIV vaccine initiative', *Press Release* WHO/UNAIDS, 21 February.

Widdus, R. (2001), 'Public-private partnerships for health: their main targets, their diversity, and their future directions', Bulletin of the World Health Organization, 2001, 79 (8), pp. 713–720.

World Bank (2002), 'River Blindness Partners Pledge $39 Million To Eliminate Disease In All Of Africa By 2010', *Press Release* 2002/152/AFR.

WTO (2002), 'Declaration on the TRIPS Agreement and Public Health', Doc. WTO 01–5770, 14 November.

Yamey, G. (2001), 'Global vaccine initiative creates inequity, analysis concludes', *British Medical Journal*.

Yamey, G. (2002), 'WHO in 2002, Faltering steps towards partnerships', *British Medical Journal*, Vol. 325, 23 November, p. 1239.

Zeitz, P.S. (2003), 'Waging a global fight more efficiently', *International Herald Tribune*, 4 March.

Index

For Product Safety Concerns and Information please contact our EU
representative GPSR@taylorandfrancis.com
Taylor & Francis Verlag GmbH, Kaufingerstraße 24, 80331 München, Germany